Praise for *When Women Get Sick*

"We all know women who have been diagnosed with cancer or serious illness or will be, and the anxiety can be paralyzing. *When Women Get Sick* is a beacon in the midst of that fear. Rebecca Bloom draws on a lifetime of compassion and twenty-five years' experience as a patient advocate to walk readers through the complex healthcare system and workplace issues, helping women advocate for themselves and their well-being. If it feels like this book came straight from her heart, you're right. This labor of love can save you immeasurable money and stress. It could even save your life."

—**Debra Engle**, executive director of Story Summit
and bestselling author of *The Only
Little Prayer You Need*

"Trust Rebecca Bloom. Her book will be your guiding angel when you are coping with a cancer diagnosis or another serious illness."

—**Delia Ephron**, screenwriter, author of *Left on
Tenth: A Second Chance at Life*

"Having the broadest lens is critical to seeing your way to the other side of a catastrophic diagnosis. Rebecca Bloom's book *When Women Get Sick* augments our collective vision to see that improvement in women's healthcare must be a holistic movement. By streamlining every level of care—from insurance to HR to diagnosis to treatment—Bloom demonstrates that remedying the injustices so many women encounter in the treatment of illness is imperative in the quest for equity writ large."

—**Amy E. Herman**, author of *Visual Intelligence: Sharpen Your Perception, Change Your Life* and *Fixed: How to Perfect the Fine Art of Problem Solving*

"If you or a woman you care about is in a health crisis, this book is your guide to how to navigate the healthcare system, the insurance system, *and* the workplace. Rebecca Bloom has written clearly and beautifully about what every woman needs to know to be successful in managing her health. This book shouldn't need to exist—but given our current environment, it has to. Thank you, Rebecca, for writing it. I will be recommending it to every woman I know."

—**Sarah McDonald**, author of *The Cancer Channel: One Year. Two Cancers. Three Miracles.*

"If we live long enough, we'll all encounter illness. Then what? Navigating women's health is complicated, as are the insurance, employer, and provider systems involved in getting the care we need, especially when facing life-threatening issues. That's where this engaging book comes in. Both angel and advocate, Rebecca Bloom offers advice that is deeply intelligent, accessible, personal—and game-changing. It will help you access the information and services you need when the stakes are high. An absolute must-read."

—**Jill Sherer Murray**, TEDx speaker and author of *Big Wild Love: The Unstoppable Power of Letting Go*

"Imagine if your lifelong best friend happened to be a top-level employee benefits lawyer and women's healthcare advocate who could navigate the deadly waters of the US healthcare system for you. Now stop imagining it and read *When Women Get Sick* by Rebecca Bloom, who will be that friend for you. Bloom shares expert insider advice on how to cut through the infuriating red tape of a healthcare system optimized for profit rather than cure. This is the kind of time-saving and lifesaving book that shouldn't be necessary in the first place, but given the shambolic state of access to decent medical care for all, it is imperative reading for women and their careers. When Bloom signs off with the words 'Count me in for the long haul. I'll walk with you,' I believe her!"

—**Gila Pfeffer**, author of *Nearly Departed: Adventures in Loss, Cancer, and Other Inconveniences*

"I wish I'd had this smart, practical, and deeply comforting book when I was thirty-seven and navigating treatment, with a young son, a growing career, and the demands of family life. Balancing chemotherapy, radiation, and the needs of my loved ones felt overwhelming, and this book provides the kind of comprehensive empowerment I desperately needed then. I'm so glad it's now available to support other women and their families on similar health journeys."

—**Anna Rathkopf**, award-winning photographer, director, cancer advocate, and author of *HER2: The Diagnosed, the Caregiver and Their Son*

"Rebecca Bloom has spent decades assisting women through the maze of concerns that arise beyond the actual medical issues—work, insurance, and legal aspects of the journey are all critical to successfully navigating this unfamiliar road. With this book, she makes her advocacy even more broadly available to those in need. Avail yourself of Rebecca's experience and expertise so you can focus your energy on healing."

—**Lynn Smolik**, MD

"*When Women Get Sick* offers a rare mix of legal savvy, practical expertise, feminist perspective—and deep humanity—to help navigate the nation's unruly trio of healthcare, employment, and benefits systems. This is a searing and eye-opening read packed with how-to advice for every imaginable scenario, and Rebecca Bloom is the women's health advocate and champion we all deserve."

—**Jennifer Weiss-Wolf**, executive director, Birnbaum Women's Leadership Network at NYU School of Law

"*When Women Get Sick* is a book no one wants to need, but many will benefit by reading. As the title correctly notes, getting sick isn't an 'if'; it's a 'when.' And yet, our healthcare system is complicated, exhausting to navigate, and nearly impossible to figure out in a moment of need. Rebecca Bloom combines insights from her experiences as a lawyer, corporate HR leader, and women's health advocate to create a much-needed guide, with creative, engaging writing that makes it an enjoyable read—as well as one I wish I'd had in my own cancer journey."

—**Sally Joy Wolf**, well-being advisor, stage IV cancer thriver, and advocate, inspirational speaker

WHEN WOMEN GET SICK

WHEN WOMEN GET SICK

AN EMPOWERING APPROACH
FOR GETTING THE SUPPORT YOU NEED

REBECCA BLOOM

Broadleaf Books
Minneapolis

WHEN WOMEN GET SICK
An Empowering Approach for Getting the Support You Need

30 29 28 27 26 25   2 3 4 5 6 7 8 9

Library of Congress Control Number: 2024950972 (print)

Cover design: Juicebox Designs

Print ISBN: 979-8-8898-3231-7
eBook ISBN: 979-8-8898-3232-4

To my mother, my sister, and my daughters.
To every daughter, sister, or mother touched by illness.
To all who love and care for them.

R.B.

CONTENTS

Introduction   ix

1. Set Yourself Up for Support   1
2. What Kind of Help to Ask For   15
3. What Can Happen at Work and How
   to Maximize Benefits   33
4. Taming the Health Insurance Beast   51
5. Even If You Have Insurance,
   Stay Prepared   67
6. Access to Advice, Diagnostics,
   and Treatment   83
7. Communicating with Your Doctors   107
8. What to Do If a Bill Is Wrong or
   Coverage Is Denied   125
9. Creative Solutions and Mindfulness   139
10. What Is the Real Problem?   155
11. The Safety Net   169
    Conclusion   187
    We Can Make This Better for Women

Acknowledgments   201
Notes   209

INTRODUCTION

I'VE BEEN TRAINING for this my whole life.

I wanted to go to law school from the time I could talk. There was a bit of an approval feedback loop, I have to say. The more I got snaps at the family dinner table for being sharp, funny, and incisive, the more I blurted out silly things like "May I approach the bench?" when asking, say, for seconds of my mother's delicious handmade challah—kneaded, as she once wrote, with "currants and hope." My dad is a lawyer and my grandfather, his father, was one too. It wasn't something my grandmothers, aunts, or even my plucky, outspoken mother considered. My maternal grandfather, for sure, was an ahead-of-his-time feminist and would have supported his firstborn, hyper-verbal, Virgo daughter, but my mother's artistic soul was destined for other things, and the lawyering on that side of the family was left to her younger brother, a Taurus whose birthday I share.

But me? Card-carrying member of the ACLU! Mock trial kid. Looker-at-all-phenomena-through-a-legal-lens. Memorizer of the speeches from *Inherit the Wind*. Get-outer-of-speeding-tickets! Reader of books like John Rawls's *A Theory of Justice* well before I could possibly comprehend what he was talking about. I'm not sure I understand it even now. But

I fell hard for the idea that there was some set of rules that we could all agree were fair and just and that could keep our social contract together, a system we could put in place to make sure that everybody got theirs, be they criminals, retirees, the disabled, or members of what lawyers call "suspect classifications." My adolescent mind was drawn in by what I saw as an elegant symmetry, rights and responsibilities, crime and punishment, costs and benefits. Somehow that felt like balance, and way before the mindfulness movement took over everyone's blog, before there even were blogs, I found this intellectually irresistible.

Here's one thing I know I believed: that it was a lawyer's job to uphold the tenets of justice. Represent your client's side to the best of your ability, sure, but with some sacred understanding that this was all a choreographed exercise in service of keeping the playing field even. Why else would they care about your character and fitness before they admitted you to the bar? With that in mind, I wended through the galaxy of ideas that was my glorious college experience on my way to a big desk with a leather-bound copy of *Black's Law Dictionary* to call my own. Thanks, Uncle Jeff (the aforementioned fellow Taurus) and Aunt Judy; it really was a great graduation gift! One I have used often.

When I started law school, there wasn't much question in my mind about what was next for me. I'd amble right on over to the Legal Aid Society, a legal organization for children, or some other perch befitting my lofty ideals, briefcase in hand, ready to join the fray and make a difference. But the reality of student loans changed my choices. And let's be clear—what I owed in total is now about what students pay for just one year of law school.

I ended up at one of the most well-known New York City law firms, three names recognizable to legal and business insiders, the power font etched in marble. To non-lawyers, they all seem the same. By the early nineties, even though the job market was tight, these firms had realized that recruiting the best and the brightest might mean expanding their hiring pool beyond white men. Today they know better still. But in those days, I would feel my female otherness when I walked into a conference room in a pink linen suit, facing down a sea of navy and pinstripe two-pieces.

I knew it wouldn't last for me. Something about the way the scent of the impeccable fresh flowers on every floor grabbed my imagination and sent me running to my office to pen short stories spelled trouble. I worked so hard. I never went to the theater, hardly saw my beloved parents, and would go years without talking to some of my friends. I was already married when I started, which was a good thing, because dating would not have happened. There just wasn't time. I figured out early that if I was going to be able to stay long enough to pay for my education without losing my marbles, I'd have to find a niche. I needed an intellectual puzzle of some kind that connected me to people, because though I liked most of the employees at my firm, I simply did not care one whit for the business interests of my firm's clients—banks, venture capital firms, and ginormous multinational corporations.

I chose a somewhat narrow path—that of employee benefits and compensation, a combination of how an employer provides for employees in terms of pay, health insurance, disability, and stock options. I had become obsessed with workplace discrimination in law school, especially age discrimination. New York State had mandatory retirement for teachers in those days, and my beloved grandfather, J. Philip Cook, the aforementioned forward-thinking feminist, had been forced to retire. When they changed the law, he went right back to teaching. But it bothered me to see a person so vibrant, energetic, and involved be treated like a number instead of an individual. So much so that I did an independent study with a brilliant labor professor about the Age Discrimination in Employment Act. I just wanted to understand how things really worked. How injustices got addressed in the real world. How wrongs were righted.

As an employee benefits and compensation lawyer, I had to become an expert in a law called *ERISA* (the Employee Retirement Income Security Act of 1974, as amended), the even less sexy cousin of the already much maligned Internal Revenue Code (we had to learn a bit about that too). Tax lawyers at these places were seen by the majority of big firm lawyers as a nerdy and necessary evil. The structurers of deals, they weren't cool like the mergers and acquisitions people, who were like the thoracic surgeons of the corporate law world—the macho elite. *ERISA* lawyers were a step down from there, the butt of many a "what *is* it that you do, exactly?" joke at the attorney teas that were held every Thursday. In exchange for this low-woman-on-the-cool-food-chain status, I thought maybe I'd have a better quality of life and learn something human-centered that might somehow feed my pilgrim soul. Neither was quite to be. A deal's a deal, and when a conglomerate is buying every packaged cookie company in the Lower 48, there are a lot of employee benefit plans to audit, people on disability to fight over (*"who takes them?"*—this is how they talk about people in corporate America), options to maybe accelerate, key employees to tie up with rich golden parachute agreements (look it up, it's gross)—in other words, there's plenty to stay up all night over! As for the complexity puzzle part? Well, yes, it was like a Sunday crossword and then some. When inappropriate talk includes phrases such as "I'd like to subordinate your debentures," I think it's safe to say there's a kind of dark grandiloquence on parade anyway. Don't get me wrong; it wasn't all bad. I met some wonderful colleagues brimming with intelligence and the integrity to match. The winner-takes-all ethos of corporate America is one thing, but people are people, and there are many good ones. Also, the high standards matched my excellence junkie tendencies. It just wasn't a fit for me forever.

About five years in, a few miraculous things happened. First and foremost, I got pregnant. That meant many things, including that I refused to take my commuter running shoes off. *Sorry, fellas. Wanna go? I'm with child. And I know the laws that protect me in this here workplace.* The mergers kept on coming, fast and furious. Days, nights, and weekends. After my baby girl was born, I contended with the truth—I was almost done paying back my student loans, and I had never known love like this. The paid maternity leave ran out. I asked for an unpaid extension of another four months. It was granted, and by the time I was ready to kiss a shot at partnership goodbye, my husband talked me into moving to the Silicon Valley, where he was being enthusiastically recruited. So we went, and the decision to walk away from corporate law was made without me having to overthink it. A few years later, my old boss called me and asked if I wanted to join their new Northern California office. I said "no, thank you" because motherhood from the get-go was consuming in a good way. I'd started my own consulting business by this time, all in the service of spending every possible second with my mesmerizing daughter. I just couldn't imagine why I would ever sign up to go back to eighty-hour work weeks. Plus, when I thought about it from a distance, I found that using my brains to make rich people richer made me awfully sad.

Speaking of rich people, we settled into a very different culture—tech, innovation, parking lot and coffee shop chit-chat about who owns what stock in what company and who is the founder of what. It was a neo–gold rush, and I felt like an alien, yet I spoke the language because of my work experience. All told, it was an odd time to be trying to find a place for myself. Then my mother was diagnosed with breast cancer back in New York, and I felt so far away.

Before I get into what happened next, I pause to provide some backstory. My beloved Aunt Esther—groundbreaking feminist, first female graduate of Yeshiva University (where she got her master's), shaker of Eleanor Roosevelt's hand, supporter of immigrants and the arts, and an all-around badass— was a breast cancer survivor. Her diagnosis and treatment happened well before the disease was understood. She had surgery. That's it. And she survived. It wasn't something we talked much about. Her husband died young, and she kept about her business as a teacher, social worker, opera lover, and social justice warrior. She puffed cigarettes but did not inhale, lived a Lincoln Center life, read voraciously, and always kept a hankie tucked inside her Speidel watchband. I came into the city whenever I could to sit with her in the front row at the New York State Theater to see whatever opera was playing. I did not love opera, but I was mad about her.

Another family member, my mother's cousin Thelma, the mother of my adored second cousins Merilee and Amy, died of breast cancer in 1979. I was twelve years old, and this loss devastated me. I remember driving up to the Catskills for the funeral, singing to myself in my head as I looked out the window through the misty rain. I could not fathom their hurt and have carried it with me always. With these loved ones in my heart, my mother's diagnosis terrified me. I began to see breast cancer as a beast, a scourge that took away mothers.

A disease that decimated families. Including mine. A new mother myself, something changed in me. I reckoned with how desperately I needed my mother and how much my daughter, Sam, needed me.

Sam and I went back to New York to be with my mother, aptly named Linda (she is so beautiful), for her surgery and her treatments, staying in my childhood home for a month and a half, memories all around. It all went as well as could be expected—my dad was still employed and insured, and she was on his plan. She got good care and went on to thrive (as I edit this introduction, it's the month of her eighty-sixth birthday). Most of the time, I guarded the door, thanking the well-wishers and accepting flowers, food, and thoughtful gifts from my mother's friends, running the point so she could rest. There were a few moments when there was more to the job. When she wasn't sure what to do next, how to get the opinions she needed, what would be covered, and why she got a certain bill. We worked it out as a family by making calls, reading and interpreting complicated things, and calling upon doctor friends to help us out. She was my father's wife, and he was a lawyer, a reader, a connector, and a skilled advocate. As was I. Together, we were dynamite, and it gave us something to focus on and tamp down our worries and stress.

I was stopped in my tracks by the question of what happens to women who don't have either that level of security or that kind of in-house team. I don't think I understood how naive a question this was when I originally asked myself.

I had no idea, but I was about to find out by beginning a professional journey with Bay Area Cancer Connections and learning from their diverse array of clients, women from all walks of life facing unique and specific challenges. It turns out, unless you have paid for incredibly high-priced concierge doctors, which generally only the very wealthy even consider, this healthcare system we have in place, particularly as it pertains to payment for services but definitely in terms of access and employment too, is designed to leave you holding the bag. It can be awful for patients. It makes people run, ignore, put off, deny, and disappear. Anything to avoid the experience of being placed on hold for hours, given the same unsatisfactory answer repeatedly by a person reading from a manual, told something is covered and then finding out it isn't when it's already too late or being made to feel like a number or a case instead of a human being whose life is worth tending to and saving.

I realized, arriving home from caring from my mother, that I had been given a gift in the form of a body of knowledge, experience in asking the right questions and skills honed from staying up all night parsing through complex things. It so happens that in my lawyer job I had learned about both the healthcare/health insurance world and the world of the workplace. *Eureka.* My own neo–gold rush. What if instead of charging an absurd amount of money to draft complicated pension documents for people getting divorces, as I was doing, I did something better in tandem with this mom dance? I thought about how I could flip the script—I knew how the big companies, insurers, and bottom-liners approached these things. I could use that information to look at it from the individual side. I could help women think it all through when they are diagnosed with cancer—there are so many questions and so few definitive answers. Unexpected challenges arise that have nothing to do with healing. And I could help. I'm a lawyer, not a doctor, but I am driven to contribute to the healing of mothers and others. To be a woman who helps save other women.

I'll never forget the day I had a meeting at an organization that was then called Community Breast Health Project in Palo Alto, California, with the then executive director. Back then, they had a small office behind a swanky lingerie store. Truly. It was and still is a patient-first support organization, full of wonderful professionals who have never lost sight of their admirable mission—to support "anyone affected by breast cancer with personalized services that inform and empower."

At the time, around 1997, they holistically helped women with breast cancer, as there were very few who lived with ovarian cancer for long. They are now called Bay Area Cancer Connections, and the mission has expanded to women with ovarian cancer as well, though I've never seen them turn anyone with any kind of health challenge away. As I said to their first executive director, "I know some things that I think might help your clients. Could we see if there's a way to leverage my experience?" That lovely woman smiled at me and said simply, "Are you kidding me?" And that's how the longest and proudest professional association of my life began—serving as a volunteer patient and workplace advocate for women with cancer, which I have been honored to do for over twenty-six years.

Though I already knew that the healthcare, coverage, and employer-provided benefits world was a jungle, I must say that my cushy corporate training did not fully prepare me for exactly how pronounced this "land of the free and the home of the you-better-not-get-sick-or-you-could-be-looking-at-financial-ruin" situation had become. It simply didn't come across that big desk.

It was incredible to me that a woman could work herself to the bone forty-plus hours a week for years and still be on the edge like that. Or that people could really be one-asthma-puffer-fifteen-years-ago away from being denied coverage. I knew about this law that was passed in the eighties called HIPAA, mostly because of its privacy rules, but I didn't realize that there was a hole you could drive an ambulance through. If you weren't on a *group* insurance plan, the preexisting condition rules that were supposed to protect people who'd been sick from losing their coverage or preventing them from getting new coverage did *not* apply to you. I couldn't believe that in the richest country in the world, this was how we did things. That issue wasn't fixed until President Obama addressed it with the Affordable Care Act of 2008. And that wasn't the half of it.

If you or a woman you care about is fighting a serious illness, this book will share the rest: the ins and outs of how to navigate the healthcare industrial complex and the workplace. Could these learnings apply to a man or a boy? Yes. The first book I worked on as a writer was entitled *Breast Cancer in the Workplace*, published by the Northern California Cancer Center through a grant from the Fisher Family after their patriarch, Gap CEO Don Fisher, had breast cancer—which men do get, though it is rare. Years later, the Cancer Prevention Institute of California reprinted the book after expanding it to cover all cancers, because the rules and lessons and practical tips for employers applied regardless of the kind of cancer or gender identification of the patient-employee. They called it *Cancer in the Workplace*, and I served as a consulting editor. Both books were designed to help employers understand the legalities and practicalities involved when their employees are diagnosed, as well as resources and information to help support them. These books were provided to employers in the state of California. This book is for the patients, and while I'm directing it at people who identify as women with serious illness, if it serves others, that's a win for the good people.

For the last twenty-six years, I have developed an abiding passion for supporting women's health. I've seen what women contend with through the eyes of the many women I've worked with, my mother's successful breast cancer battle, my sister facing down the disease, as well as scares, surgeries, tests, and preventive measures I have gone through myself. I mean to give you the tools to make this a less lonely and con- fusing experience and share the stories of other women. To help you not go bankrupt, lose your professional identity, san- ity, or security while getting through cancer or another serious illness. This isn't a political tome; it's a practical, story-filled survival guide. No one person or one organization can top- ple a system alone—not that I won't continue to try and link arms with others who wish we could. But in the meantime, my sense for any woman dealing with cancer or another seri- ous illness is that it is better to know than not to know. To be empowered in every possible way. To be gifted a pair of pitfall goggles. I know it's atrocious that we need a bag of tricks to get proper care in this country when we are sick without fac- ing financial ruin or a mental health event. But if this is what we're stuck with, I want to help.

Our system makes it clear what our societal values are, and they do not prioritize women's wellness. Women's healthcare and control of women's bodies has been in the crosshairs of perhaps the most prolonged culture war in history. The best you can do today is learn the tools of self-advocacy. And the best I can do is walk beside you as a woman trying to help other women.

Nobody should need a book like this. And I look forward to a day when our country becomes civilized to the point that nobody will. In the meantime, I hope what's here will help.

R.B.

〔 1 〕

Set Yourself Up for Support

I'M SAD TO say I've seen similar versions of the story I'll share next too many times. It goes something like this: A hardworking woman gets married or partners with another person and has kids. She makes some compromises, because raising kids is a harder and more expensive endeavor than ever before. So, she creates a solution, taking hard-earned skills and becoming a consultant or moving to gig work. It seems like a smart choice, giving her more flexibility and possibly higher hourly pay; maybe she is even in the enviable position of having a partner who has health insurance and other benefits, so she doesn't need to duplicate them. I did this myself, and I don't regret it when I think of all the experiences I had with my now-adult daughters that I might have missed out on. I'm also aware that I gave up status, security, and earning potential when I made that choice.

This staple-it-together way to raise a family can be great, especially if you stay married. But divorce happens with predictable frequency.[1] For women, this is true in hetero and same-sex marriages. I'm reminded specifically of the day that I was asked to call a woman named Alicia. Alicia's marriage had unofficially broken up a few years before. She and her partner had never filed any paperwork or hammered out a separation agreement. They just were going along, figuring it out. People are wary of the "divorce machine," its costs and stressors. Having consulted for divorce lawyers myself, I cannot blame them. There are many junctures that can cause unexpected disputes that generate big legal bills. Alicia had three kids and two part-time jobs. Her not-yet-ex-wife was a decent person; they just wanted different things for their futures, and though it was sad and hard, it wasn't contentious. Alicia's partner intended to keep the kids on her health insurance, provided by her big tech employer, and didn't mind keeping Alicia on the plan while the matter was still pending. They don't make movies like *Kramer vs. Kramer* about families like this, but it's often the way things work. Good, slightly heartbroken people trying to do as right by one another as they can.

Alicia and her partner decided to move ahead and file some paperwork after they'd been living apart for some time, with a peaceful co-parenting and financial support situation already in place. They agreed it would be easier and better for their kids, and there really wasn't much left to discuss. They felt they'd figured it out. They saved time, money, and heartache—what we call nowadays a "conscious uncoupling."[2] Once Alicia's partner's employer figured out that the marriage was over, they took her off her partner's policy. The carriers require this. Nothing nefarious on anyone's part. Just people and organizations following the rules.

Alicia didn't anticipate what happened next. She bought what she thought was a reasonable Affordable Care Act policy from her state exchange, and just about six months later, she found out she had breast cancer. Fortunately for her, the policy she had purchased was accepted by her local medical system—at first. For the initial three months of her treatment, which included many appointments, imaging, and the start of chemotherapy, she was able to see the doctors she wanted to see in the same place she'd given birth to her babies and taken them for all their needs as they grew. But then, that system dropped her new plan. She was given a few months' notice, but that did not save her from stress. It wasn't that the upcoming treatments and surgery themselves were suddenly not covered at all by the plan; it was that she was faced with the choice of going out of network and paying more out of pocket for the care team that had been recommended by doctors she already knew and trusted or starting over. Because the costs for these now out-of-network doctors looked exorbitant, she started over in a new system, a farther drive away and separate from the group of medical professionals that treated the rest of her family. This was destabilizing. It affected her mental health and, consequently, her recovery. But newly single and now on her own in terms of health insurance, she had no other viable choice.

A gracious person, Alicia still counted herself as one of the lucky ones, and she had a point. When it comes to divorce and financial marginalization, there are stories of acrimonious battles, impossible choices, and financial wipeouts. Women lose health insurance after marital disruption not only through the loss of a partner's coverage but also indirectly, because they get stuck not being able to afford or access other coverage. The federal law known as COBRA (Consolidated Omnibus Budget Reconciliation Act of 1985) gives former spouses an option to purchase an extension of the coverage they had with their spouse for up to thirty-six months in some cases (eighteen in others), but premiums are usually somewhere between high and stratospheric. Even though many women sustain major economic setbacks after divorce, few become eligible for subsidies or Medicaid. They get stuck in the middle. Medicare serves the elderly and disabled, and because a larger percentage of divorces happen before retirement age and the disability qualification is limited, it is seldom an option.[3] Alicia had an extremely stressful experience because of insurance changes necessitated by her divorce. These kinds of experiences are likely to happen to more women if unbridled greed continues to win the day inside of the medical-industrial complex.

In these situations, the best defense for women is to line up the right kinds of support. In all arenas, women deserve champions and access to quality information, especially when the stakes are their physical and emotional wellness and financial security.

Proactivity Is Key

Nobody plans for a serious diagnosis. When it comes, it is often accompanied by shock, pain, denial, fear, and anger. That doesn't feel like an optimal moment to engage in planning, and yet clearly thinking ahead is what eases the journey. This is a challenge given all that swirls around at such a difficult moment. Years of supporting women at this painful point have taught me what works and how to express those learnings. Like most things worth doing, it is layered and takes energy.

Think through Insurance Coverage

The best way to start is with targeted proactivity. The first line of business is health insurance, or at least a plan for how any necessary treatments, surgeries, or medications will be paid for. We'll cover insurance in more detail in chapter 4, but for now let me emphasize this: comprehensive healthcare coverage is not just nice to have. It's self-care table stakes in an ever-complicated world. It goes well before Instagrammable vacations and cable, just after food, clothing, and shelter. This is the case not only for a woman's loved ones but for herself. Women should not "make due" when it comes to healthcare coverage. There are other places to cut corners or to prioritize other people, especially kids, but health coverage is not the place. If you find yourself with a diagnosis, check in immediately with the administrators in your doctors' offices about the coverage you have. If you need to purchase coverage, find out what they accept. If you are low-income and have not explored Medicaid policies, get right on it. Many people end up with better coverage this way than through an inexpensive plan with a high deductible, high copayments, or one that is not widely accepted. Another thing to consider if coverage is hard to find or too expensive is the services that are available at the county hospitals in your area. Many hospitals treat people for free, but check in immediately with hospital personnel to learn what that looks like. These hospitals may have longer wait times for certain treatments, but they are nonetheless viable options to consider, depending on the circumstances.

This is a great place to emphasize that every situation is different. To get this right, it pays to pay attention. You may find yourself with an unaggressive or degenerative illness, which might mean to you that being treated immediately is not your first priority, and that perhaps you'd prefer to wait for a specific doctor or clinic that is a leader in what you're dealing with. Or you could learn that fast action is warranted—and that, too, can color the way you think about accessing medical care with the best coverage possible. Part of thinking ahead is analyzing what's most important to you based on your diagnosis, financial circumstances, responsibilities, and mental state. They all figure in the equation.

What Proactivity Looks Like in the Workplace

The second aspect of proactivity is thinking through your work situation if you're employed. We'll get into more about what can happen at work when a woman gets sick in chapter 3, but a top-line consideration is the laws that may apply to provide standards and safe harbors for reasonable accommodation, leaves of absence, and other protections that employees count on when they get sick. Available employee benefits are the other main avenue to mine. In a nutshell, be aware. Think about where you work and what that means. A school is not the same thing as a start-up, and a nonprofit is different from a multinational corporation. All entities have their advantages, whether it's financial wherewithal or flexibility. They each have unique pressures and priorities too.

If you've not done it beforehand, at the point of a diagnosis, take stock of your employee benefits, regardless of whether you're at the executive or entry level. You might have suddenly accessible retirement funds, paid leaves, life insurances policies that pay disability benefits, and other programs available to you that will be useful as you navigate your health situation. The law requires that most employers give out employee handbooks or have them available online. Most employees never read them. They aren't entertaining, but they are information-rich. One of my first jobs out of law school involved writing them, so I'm keenly aware of this. Finding out what your benefits are, what your workplace options look like, and which protective laws apply to you is always a good idea.

I often tell women I work with that these protections and benefits are not giveaways and using them is not accepting charity. They are part of being an employee. You've earned them. If you need to access state or federal disability programs, these are not a gift to you either. You've paid into the system. So many women are conditioned to be givers that you'd be surprised how much they need to hear this.

Why Advocacy Is So Important for Women

A friend recently told me that her feminist daughter had the wry idea that if she ever does a gender reveal party, she'd go for the sealed envelope approach. If it's a boy, inside the envelope will be a dollar bill, but if it's a girl then the envelope will contain eighty-two cents. When it comes to healthcare in America, women are similarly short-changed. When a woman faces down the medical-industrial complex, historical inequalities present challenges that radiate. Much has been written about the persistent gender inequality in the health space and the workplace. From pay gaps to medical research, strides have been made but there are miles to go.

Knowing the facts about what women face is the first step in working toward more affordable, accessible healthcare and fairness in the workplace. For starters, women are more likely than men to be unemployed, underemployed, or under-resourced.

This is a complicated sociological issue, and while the way we live and arrange ourselves in households has changed over time,[4] one thing that has remained the same is that women, particularly women of color, are more likely to be economically marginalized than men.[5] This isn't new. Barbara Ehrenreich's groundbreaking book, *Nickel and Dimed: On (Not) Getting By in America*, came out in 2001.[6] It was a look back on the Welfare Reform Act of 1966 and its effects on the working poor. And long before we were talking about the sacrifices of front-line and essential workers in the age of COVID-19, it argued that low-wage workers were getting a raw deal in America and we were all living off their generosity, not the other way around.

Because women are far more likely to struggle financially than men, many aspects of their health journeys are affected. Here's a hard truth: nearly 70 percent of low-wage workers in America are women. It doesn't take much extrapolation to see why women would have so much to lose compared to men when they get sick. These jobs have less flexibility, fewer benefits, and more turnover by nature. In the United States, only 21 percent of low-wage employees have paid sick leave.[7] Additionally, 40 percent of low-wage workers work for small businesses (as compared with 20 percent of all workers). Federal laws such as the Americans with Disabilities Act and the Family Medical Leave Act don't apply to small businesses (under fifteen or fifty employees, respectively), which excludes these employees from their protections. Workers who are off the books, such as many domestic employees, may not have significant employee benefits to fall back on either.[8] Since women are more likely to be poor than men even if they are employed, healthcare costs are quite likely to threaten their economic security. If they're working in low-wage jobs, they will face both flexibility issues and affordability challenges— they may not have paid sick time, and taking time off to get care may be difficult if not impossible. Consequently, they are much more vulnerable to losing their jobs when they get sick. Women struggle with medical bills and debt at a higher incidence than men. In 2016, one in four women surveyed reported difficulty paying medical bills.[9]

To add to this brew, women need more healthcare than men over their lifetimes, which is attributable to several factors. Women are more likely to have chronic conditions, use prescription drugs, and battle depression. Additionally, regardless of whether they have children, women interact more with medical professionals during their reproductive years.[10]

The Affordable Care Act has been weakened. When Congress eliminated the buy-in mandate and attendant tax penalty, more healthy Americans opted out. Without a large risk and cost-sharing pool, prices have increased and plans in state marketplaces are simply less affordable. Some women go uninsured because they don't qualify for Medicaid, but they still cannot afford individual policies and are not eligible for group policies. In 2021, 64 percent of uninsured adults reported that they were uninsured because the cost of coverage was too high.[11] Many women do not have access to coverage through a job or a partner, and some, notably poor women in states that did not expand Medicaid, are ineligible for financial assistance for coverage. Additionally, undocumented immigrants are ineligible for Medicaid or Marketplace coverage.[12]

On average, women have lower incomes than men and have been more likely to qualify for Medicaid.[13] However, during the 2016–2020 Trump administration, there were cutbacks to Medicaid that included new rules allowing states to institute work requirements, based on the false narrative that Medicaid enrollees are taking advantage of free healthcare and not working to remain eligible.[14] None of this is simple, but taken as a whole, our political reality and the complicated healthcare laws and the incentives they create hurt women disproportionately. Systemic change is needed. The status quo simply isn't working for many women. Women need support, and often, they will get it from advocates.

When a woman gets sick, whether she's is a gig worker or an executive, it's overwhelming. Women have more in common than there are abstractions that separate us, and every woman deserves support—a person (or people) she can count on to help her untangle it all. Someone to listen, ask questions, and challenge assumptions. It's practical, but psychologically important too. Connection is a well-documented social determinant of health. A doctor friend of mine who specializes in breast surgery made it very clear to me that advocacy changes women's attitudes and paves the way for better healing. The age of the advocate is upon us.

TIPS AND TAKEAWAYS

Regardless of employment or financial status, there are ways for every woman facing illness to set herself up to be supported. With the right guidance, every woman facing cancer or another serious illness can do some smart planning and be empowered.

Not everyone will have all the healthcare options or workplace benefits and flexibility available. But here are some high-level tips for each arena to bear in mind. There will be much more about health insurance, how to get it, keep it, and maximize coverage—as well as how to take advantage of workplace benefits and other work-related issues—in later chapters.

IN THE HEALTH SPACE

Before Diagnosis

Choose your policy wisely. Whether you have an individual or employer-provided policy, you will have an open enrollment period every year. Check deductibles, out-of-pocket maximums, and most importantly, whether the policy is accepted by the doctors you're most likely to use.

Hang on to the paperwork or know where to find the details online. You will want to know the rules of your policy, such as copayments in- and out-of-network, need for preapproval of care, and exclusions that may apply. Knowing these things in advance of getting care can save you money, time, and aggravation.

Once Diagnosed

Shopping around for the best price and coverage for a proce-dure, diagnostics, or ongoing care makes good sense. Check your health insurance online portal for tools that will help you explore fair pricing.

Before you agree to care with a provider, find out if they are in-network, which will be more affordable for you. This includes specialists such as radiologists, anesthesiologists, and pathologists. Ask before you undergo treatment or procedures. This is by far the best way to avoid unforeseen bills.

Check your health insurance website for special dis-counts on programs and benefits that may be useful to you in your health journey. There are often nutrition programs, lifestyle options such as yoga or meditation, and other groups and classes that may help you.

Spend some time finding out about disease-specific orga-nizations that support patient journeys. Often, these organi-zations are set up to fill the gaps and help you find lower-cost or free solutions for things like prosthetics, alternative healing, and other services that can help you move forward.

IN THE WORKPLACE

Find out if your employer provides sick time. If they do, what does the policy state? For some it will be a requisite number of days. For others, sick leave will be folded into paid time off and can be a requisite number of days or unlimited. Either way, you'll need to understand how it works.

Assess the size of your employer so that you can determine the basic state and federal laws that protect you. These will include laws covering leaves of absence, the availability of continued health coverage if your employment ends, antidiscrimination, and disability. You can learn more at usa.gov/workplace-laws. Search the workplace laws that are applicable in your state or city.

Ask for access to an online or hard copy form of your employee handbook so that you can read about the benefits that your employer provides. These can include health insurance, life insurance, flexible spending plans, short- and long-term disability, and retirement plans.

❨ 2 ❩

What Kind of Help to Ask For

RARELY DOES A true genius walk into your world or your Zoom living room. This happened to me while teaching a writing workshop. I was the leader and facilitator of the group, but I learned so much from Sarah, her mind-blowing work, and her creative storytelling abilities. When I realized that she was struggling with a serious and not-yet-fully-understood illness, I got worried. She is an award-winning playwright and performer who waited tables for decades to support her creative work and connect with people. Covid shut down the in-person restaurant business in New York City, where she lives. Knowing this sent my patient and workplace advocate brain into overdrive. I became concerned about Sarah's income, health insurance, mental health, and overall security as soon as she let on that she was not well. I am too familiar with how this constellation of issues can hurt a woman.

I decided to overstep my writing teacher boundaries and ask Sarah about her insurance circumstances, medical team, and income replacement situation. These are strangely intimate questions because of laws that protect our financial and health information.[1] Still, when you think of the ways people give away their data and personal information on social media, it's interesting that I felt sheepish asking her, but I've been trained. An open book, Sarah gave me the news. She was terrified and unsure of exactly what she was facing. When she first applied for unemployment, a smart and resourceful unemployment counselor in New York City had guided her toward a Medicaid plan in tandem with the unemployment benefits she was able to collect when the restaurant where she'd worked for years shuttered. This was a random stroke of luck, because there's simply no way that the unemployment benefits she received would have covered the COBRA premiums that Sarah was likely told about when she first lost her job. She would have been forced to look for a cheaper individual policy without any guarantee that the coverage would be comprehensive enough. Because she lives in New York City, it is unclear how affordable such a plan would have been. By the time I entered the picture, her unemployment funds had already run out, but Sarah still had the Medicaid plan. She told me that she was worried she would lose her coverage, and that she really didn't understand what the terms or duration of her plan were. She knew her insurance card had an expiration date, and she was afraid to call and ask the carrier for more information. Making these calls can be scary and confusing, and women avoid it when they are already concerned about their health. They know they will be put on hold, and they don't have confidence that they will get definitive answers.

Unfortunately, when I called the carrier, I learned that the plan did have a rapidly approaching end date. It caused Sarah considerable stress and fear when I told her because she knew she was contending with a significant health crisis. I wanted to dig deeper. Sarah probably thought it was odd that her friend and writing mentor was pleading to help her because she did not know the healthcare advocate side of me. It took her some time to adjust to the notion that I would gladly do research, get on the phone again, and try to get more answers about her Medicaid plan and what other options might be available to her in New York. The health of a wonder woman was at stake. While I already cared deeply about Sarah, I feel this way anytime I learn of a woman struggling through an illness within our challenging system.

All Women Deserve an Advocate

Humanitarian Dr. Paul Farmer beautifully said, "The idea that some lives matter less is the root of all that is wrong with the world,"[2] and this thought inspires me like no other. Every woman is worthy of a champion.

When a woman gets sick, she becomes a different person. No matter how brilliant, experienced, or resilient she is, the level of vulnerability brought to bear when facing down the medical-industrial complex is enough to make any grown woman cry. On top of that, if a woman is employed, she's going to be concerned about her job, benefits, and future prospects if she needs time off to heal or even just flexibility to be treated. None of this is simple. No matter what you've experienced or how smart you are, cancer or other serious illness can be overwhelming.

In every instance, women who get sick can benefit from an advocate: an adviser, phone caller, paper filer, close reader, researcher, sounding board, and all-around get-it-done person. Recently, I worked with a woman who is a detail-oriented financial planner with a new diagnosis. She told me that as accustomed as she is to reading the fine print and filling out forms, her experience with the healthcare system still feels like a foreign language to her because of how high and personal the stakes are. I often tell clients to tell their friends to skip the lasagna drop-off and break out the index cards, loose-leaf notebook, and scanner. What a woman who gets sick needs more than an overstuffed freezer is a chief of staff to project manage healing. On the workplace front this is important too; when a woman gets sick, she's going to have a lot of questions for human resources, department heads, and others. She's going to want to understand what her basic rights are, how she can maximize income, and what to do about sharing or guarding her medical information. There's a lot to it. If you're the person who needs someone like this, this chapter is going to give you information about exactly what to ask for. If you're the main source of someone's support, it will help you to help.

Resourcefulness and Patience Are Crucial

Finding answers and a path for Sarah took patience. The New York City system is layered, to say the least, but I used to live and practice law there, so I was not exactly a stranger to being put on hold, asking a litany of questions, writing everything down, getting disconnected, trying again, and navigating the frustrating rabbit holes that are the hallmarks of bureaucracy. My research told me there were supposed to be automatic Medicaid coverage extensions put into place for people who remained unemployed after Covid, but the system wasn't updated, and it looked, by all accounts, as though Sarah's coverage was going to expire. I found an article on a local government site that alluded to a possible extension without need for reapplication for Medicaid plans because of the pandemic, but there were no numbers to call and no follow-up steps listed. All I could find was a complicated and likely out-of-date online interface to apply and requalify. It took over five phone calls and quite a few woman hours. I scrawled names, numbers, plan information, and other details in pink ink on yellow pads and finally got to the bottom of it all, making sure I had accurate information recorded. Sarah told me she did not understand how anyone could tolerate the confusion, complexity, and stress. And that's the point. When you're facing an illness, what the system asks of us to get what we need is intolerable. Which is why finding a person—or better yet a team of people—dedicated to helping you is so crucial.

After the Medicaid renewal drama resolved, Sarah made some phone calls to her insurer and was sent to a clinic in her neighborhood. She was assured that they would accept her coverage. But it quickly became evident that this clinic did not have the resources or specialists she needed to diagnose, much less treat, her multifactorial and mysterious illness. This twist-and-turn dynamic is common. When women are fighting illness, they go from what feels like one scary episode to the next. First the securing or keeping of coverage if that is even an option, then access to care and diagnostics, then the interpreting of results and wrangling the communication and scheduling required to get treatment.

Always Be Ready to Ask

I offered to write to a childhood friend who had long served as the chief clinical officer of a large branch of one of New York's major medical systems to see if they would treat her, but Sarah was humble and hesitant about leveraging that kind of favor. I know that this kind of help isn't available to many people, but there are other ways to get to the decision-makers and get assistance that some people may not know about. For example, women's health centers and disease-specific organizations almost always have advisory boards made up of leading doctors, nurses, and hospital or medical system officials. Reaching out to these organizations can get women connected to the care and resources they need in their communities in a more efficient way than by calling or trying to make appointments online. But so many women are conditioned not to ask for this kind of help or to brush it off as unnecessary when it is offered, as though they do not feel important enough to warrant the effort. For so long, women have not been empowered to advocate for themselves in the health space or the workplace. Frustration, fear, and stress keep women from asking for what they need; it's like one of those endless games of hand over hand. This default to an antiquated norm costs us, as this is exactly the time and place to speak up. It can make a difference.

Sarah's condition worsened, and she had some unsettling and unclear tests results after waiting months for a routine procedure. At the clinic, she asked for and was denied imaging that could have uncovered answers. In a few doctors' post-appointment notes, she was called *hysterical* and *anxious,* the oldest trope in the book.[3] As though being noticeably upset was not a rational response to the Gordian knot she was facing. She was told in no uncertain terms by doctors and nurses at her clinic that there was no way her insurance would cover the imaging she had asked for, though our outside research told us that the imaging could have provided clues or answers as to what might be going on. Luckily, another of my dearest friends is an infectious disease doctor in another state who treats only Medicare and Medicaid patients. Though I did not think Sarah's condition was directly in the doctor's wheelhouse, it did involve some peripherally related body systems, so I called on her for advice. Her answers alarmed me. She told me that Sarah absolutely needed sophisticated imaging, expert specialists, multiple body system workups, and immediate attention that she was not getting.

"Rebecca," she said to me, "this could be serious." She urged me to do whatever I could to find Sarah different doctors and even spent time compiling some names she knew. She suggested that I do anything I could to get Sarah seen inside one of New York City's major medical systems and assured me that there were some doctors in places like that who would accept Medicaid. I freaked out. I called Sarah and her partner. Thank goodness they graciously and gratefully accepted my offer to get in touch with the chief clinical officer this time. I was upset but thought help might be attainable.

My friend did not disappoint. I asked him to connect Sarah immediately to the right specialists in the system he ran. He wasted no time finding her the best doctors who would accept her Medicaid plan and see her quickly. This information would not have been easy to figure out on our own. Plans get dropped routinely both by individual doctors and major medical systems, and often doctors' websites say that they accept certain plans when, in fact, they no longer do. The help of a person on the inside of the system with more knowledge than what was available to the public was invaluable. With an integrated information system now available, Sarah and her new doctors were able to rule out some of the more terrifying possibilities and connect with a medical team to support her wellness. It was dramatic, because some of the early test results looked potentially grim, especially without the added context that additional testing and imaging provided. Sarah felt cared for in a new way, like a group of experts finally had her back.

As I mentioned, the kind of help I was able to find for Sarah might seem out of reach to many, but through organizations connected to local doctors and medical professionals, it can be more accessible than people realize. Through my work with Bay Area Cancer Connections, I've called on advisory board members who are doctors when I'm helping a client who cannot get seen quickly or needs a second opinion and found them to be willing and effective resources. Clients have gotten appointments and answers through this channel. The reason that medical professionals sit on these boards is to help patients navigate the complexity that they know exists.

There is a lot to glean from this story, and I'm honored that Sarah agreed to let me write about it, because we both feel that if more women had the right advocacy in place, they could get better, faster care when it matters. To begin with, everybody needs a point person. A trusted, competent, super organized friend, sister, or neighbor. A chief of staff.

Find a Point Person, Draft Your Team

Once you find this person, think about what you need based on the specifics of your situation and your own strengths and weaknesses. For some people, it's all about the appointments.

The stressors of illness can impede concentration and make it hard to process the information you hear sitting in a doctor's office. Having someone there to listen closely while your doctor talks, and either take notes or remember key points for you, might be the balm that soothes you and keeps you focused. Additionally, this person can help you compile facts in advance and then make sure you ask your key questions. It's so easy to forget or become flustered, and women, conditioned to please, are more apt than men to worry about taking too much of a doctor's time. In today's world of electronic files, your chief of staff can log in to the portal for you, check your test results, read the doctor's notes, and help you make and calendar your follow-up appointments. Often, your test results will be posted in your portal well before your doctor reviews them and certainly before they call you to talk about them. Your point person can read the results, look up the obscure words for you, and figure out what questions the findings raise. Then, when you do connect with your doctor, you will be able to make sure your concerns are addressed. When you're stressed out, going on an Internet odyssey is rarely recommended. There's too much information/misinformation out there, and unless you are a doctor, you may not want to draw conclusions based on a study or statistic that you see in print until you know more. It can be difficult to know if what you are seeing is the most updated information, or if your case is analogous to what you are reading. An errant word or out-of-context percentage can send you around the bend, but a supportive advocate can help you stay calm while you wait to hear from your doctor.

If your condition requires that you have procedures or surgeries, your support team can help you manage visitors and communicate with friends and family to keep them informed so you can rest and be mindful about your needs. As I discuss below in the TIPS AND TAKEAWAYS section regarding drafting your team, you may need more than one person to help you cover these bases. While that may sound daunting at first, everything in life is about asking the right person, and itemizing the help you're likely to need will reveal who those people are. When they find out you're fighting an illness, friends and neighbors are likely to say "let me know what you need," and having a list of specific asks at the ready will help you take them up on their kind offers. Your chief of staff can help organize a group of caring people to give you the best support possible and match them to what you actually need. Give her a whistle and a clipboard while you get to the business of healing.

The Kind of Help You Need

This book will go into details about other ways that your team can help you along the way. Often, bills will arrive that are confusing, inflated, or just plain wrong. Just hand that bill over. Your team can make the calls, file the appeals, talk to the billing departments, fill out the forms, and send the emails.

There will be more on this topic in chapter 4, but if I had a dollar for every dollar women pay when they are wrongly charged because clearing it up is so cumbersome, I'd be a major philanthropist. I wish I could say that people don't lose their insurance or their jobs while battling illness, but it happens sometimes. This will be covered later as well, but the team who has been on the journey with you all along is often the best option to help you with these challenges if they arise.

Another thing that your team can do for you is monitor the medical journals for new studies and trials. This can be as simple as setting up a Google search that sends an email anytime there is a new development. Doctors will sometimes reach out to patients to tell them about promising new medications, procedures, or protocols, but things change quickly and doctors have pressures to treat the patients in front of them. Your trusted advocate can be of great help in this arena, even if it is just by starting a proactive dialogue with your doctor about new possibilities. After my brave and beautiful sister, Ellen, had already completed chemotherapy and surgery, a study came out about a new medication, Herceptin, that was being used for the type of breast cancer she had been diagnosed with, and the early statistics were excellent. Her oncologist called her and helped her to arrange for a year of infusions even though she was no longer in active treatment. She was relieved to have the option. This spurred me to check in with a few clients from Bay Area Cancer Connections whom I had helped because I remembered that they had been treated for the same type of breast cancer. If they had still been receiving chemotherapy, their doctors would have likely recommended the new protocol, but they hadn't heard about Herceptin. They reached out to their doctors immediately and were able to receive the treatment. This might not have happened if they had not asked.

My dear friend Sarah's situation hasn't fully resolved as of this writing, but she's gotten some promising news and some clues about what she may be dealing with. She has a team of doctors treating her, providing tests, information, procedures, and coordinated care. She recently had a surgery that may give her some relief. Things may not be perfect, but they're better. There have been other hiccups, such as the system dropping the Medicaid plan that she originally had. Thankfully, I kept files and retraced my steps and the pink ink on the yellow pad. With only two phone calls and some targeted Internet research I was able to get her onto another carrier's Medicaid plan so that she can seamlessly continue her journey back to health.

When women find themselves in scary medical situations without access to the care and coverage they need, we should all stand at attention. Women's wellness is a measure of civility, a key to a healthy society. While I do not believe we have the political will in this country for the seismic systemic changes it would take to fix this forever and for all, I do believe that there are ways to address these problems for women and others from within. It all starts with communication and compassion, with people caring for one another, standing shoulder to shoulder, advocating and navigating. Organizations like the Patient Advocate Foundation are doing remarkable work to share information and train volunteers to provide one-on-one personal advocate services to patients battling serious diseases. PAF advocates help patients work through insurance denials and healthcare access issues challenges brought on by medical debt.

It's time to create a new normal that breaks down the wall of impossibility, and organizations like PAF are leading the way. Because of the specific challenges that women face in the workplace and the health space, they especially require and deserve comprehensive advocacy.

TIPS AND TAKEAWAYS

Not every woman has access to an experienced patient advocate, and even fewer people know someone who can help them on the workplace side of things. But over years of working with women with breast and ovarian cancer, I've developed a "draft your team" approach that I share with clients regularly. Finding the right people to support your journey will set you on your way.

If you're lucky enough to have a doctor, lawyer, project manager, nurse, or human resources professional in your life, keep them in mind for the questions they may be best able to answer and consider if this person might make a good chief of staff.

When you think about the right choice for your chief of staff, be thoughtful and strategic. Competent, organized, and calm are excellent attributes to start with. If you have a partner, it may be best to ask that person for emotional support only. It's stressful to watch your loved one go through an illness. On the other hand, some people need the distraction.

Consider reaching out to an organization like the Patient Advocate Foundation or a disease-specific organization. This can help you get connected with resources and people trained to help as you build your team.

Once you find your chief of staff, here's a list of the kinds of people you might draft for your team:

- Nurse navigators at hospitals
- Social workers or patient advocates who work in the medical system where you are being treated
- Advisers at women's health organizations
- Disability/workplace experts
- Administrators and assistants in doctors' offices and healthcare centers
- Case managers at insurers
- Human resources people at your place of employment (or your partner's place of employment if you are covered under their plan)
- Neighbors who can be counted on for rides, childcare, and help with food

- Friends in the medical field who are willing to help answer basic questions or help you understand confusing vocabulary after hours
- Peers who have been through or are going through a similar journey

Once you have a chief of staff, you should work together to reach out to your wish list of potential team members. You will probably already know some of these people, but others you may need some help identifying. I have found that communicating before there is a specific problem or question is effective. Here's a sample email that you can email use:

Dear _____,

I wanted to connect with you as I embark upon a health journey that I have recently learned about. I have a feeling there may be questions that arise for me that you may be able to help me with, or there may be other ways I might hope to rely on you. Would it be alright if I reach out to you when and if questions come up?

This works well because then there's a pathway already established for cordial communication. It's so much better than a cold call at the eleventh hour.

You can always be more specific depending upon your feelings about privacy or your relationship with the people you're writing to and what you hope they can deliver.

You may run into people concerned about privacy either in the health space or the workplace if your chief of staff is the one communicating on your behalf, but in either case you can sign waivers or authorize communication on your behalf more informally. Generally, employers and medical entities will have those documents available. These are straightforward, often one-pagers that essentially have you, as a patient or employee, authorizing a medical system or employer to disclose your information to a third party of your choosing. They allow you to bring people to your appointments and help your team communicate with doctors and your employer, empowering your team to help you. Usually, these documents will be specific about the information that can be shared, such as diagnoses and prescribed medications, and will describe the purpose of the disclosure and any applicable time limits. When you're a patient on a health journey, there are so many documents you'll be given to read and sign. These will enable your team to help support you with the rest of them.

❴ 3 ❵

What Can Happen at Work
and How to Maximize Benefits

YEARS BACK, I got a call from Stephanie, a specialized software engineer and coder who worked for a big tech company. She'd been on disability during a serious illness for nine months. She was planning to return to her job, which her company had not backfilled, probably in part because her skill set was rare and she had significant expertise. She communicated to her manager that she was planning to return to work part-time at the end of the tenth month and would be able to return full-time by the end of the twelfth according to her doctors. But her manager's response was that they had hoped to find a temporary replacement sooner for her and finally had a candidate who they were bringing on. They told her she could apply for another role within the company or they could reassign her, but the only roles available were not only less senior but outside her specialized field.

Stephanie was angry and confused. As she understood it, this employer had been on her side all those months, rooting for her recovery and looking forward to welcoming her back.

Her reactions were more than understandable. She asked me what I thought were the best ways to move ahead. Spending money and time on legal advice to figure out whether this was on the wrong side of the legal line was an option for her, but she quickly saw that it would sidetrack her. The relevant question was whether she wanted to fight for her job and if she would want to stay with the company if it meant finding a different position. I asked her to decide so we could drive toward that result by communicating clearly. Stephanie decided that she only wanted her original job and team. Otherwise, she preferred to look for another position elsewhere so she could resume her career arc in her specialty field.

With that intention established, we strategized how to communicate. She told her contact in human resources that she intended to be back part-time the next month and could resume full-time a few months later, making it clear that she valued her team and colleagues and remained passionate about the work. Stephanie also said that she was not comfortable with the uncertainty or potential fit for her if their choice was to reassign her or ask her to apply for other roles. Without saying the word "demotion," she made her point. Stephanie heard back a few days later that her manager had chosen not to go with the other candidate and was looking forward to her return, even asking if there was anything they could do to ease the transition. Here, the antidiscrimination laws were a shield for Stephanie, but she did not need to rely on them as a sword. Most likely, her manager ran the communications past company lawyers and they put a stop to the hiring process because of the optics of the situation. No employer wants a lawsuit or press coverage like that. It's terrible for public relations, and in a world of social media and job application sites that include employer ratings, it is simply too much of a risk for many employers to take. Stephanie was happily surprised by the way the events unfolded, but she only stayed on an additional year because the experience soured her. She moved on to a position befitting her experience with the right title because she communicated well, stayed practical, and protected herself.

As a former workplace lawyer on the company side, I know how employers think and how decisions get made. It's often about costs and staying on the right side of the law, but it tends to be more nuanced and economy-dependent than that—in good times, employers do more to retain people, plain and simple. In leaner times, they may not try as hard. On the employee side, most women work because they need money, purpose, identity, and fulfillment, but it's also often a matter of access to benefits, particularly health insurance. Employment and insurance are hopelessly tangled because of our third-party payer system and the lack of universal healthcare in America. The result of these forces is that most employers provide health insurance coverage to their employees. In our late-capitalist society, profit is the priority and pennies get pinched, but a host of complicated laws have been designed to keep companies in check and elevate the protection of employees as they find themselves in difficult situations. Regulatory systems have also been put in place to protect members of historically relegated groups, including women and people of color.

When sick women struggle with their employers, they sometimes think about lawsuits. Well-meaning friends and family will often jump in with words like *discriminatory, greedy, evil, soulless, heartless.* While there are instances of greed and discrimination, reality tends to be more complicated. Companies and organizations are made up of individuals; mostly human beings who love other people, who have mothers, wives, sisters, and daughters. Most of the time, I have found that when a woman who is fighting an illness has challenges with her employer, the productive path is practical as opposed to strictly legal.

The key is to communicate well with the other people involved. A woman's energy is nearly always better spent on healing and self-care, as opposed to a ride on the emotional rollercoaster. Keeping it civil and productive is the top-line goal, and staying away from courts and lawyers is almost always the best course of action. Barriers to bringing lawsuits are myriad—they take a long time to settle and are quite difficult to win, even when moral outrage is well-founded. Companies spend millions of dollars setting up internal systems that allow them to make business decisions without running afoul of the law. They know how to take actions that may seem unfair but are nonetheless probably not lawsuit losers.

What constitutes "illegal" action is not usually a cut-and-dried question. Most of the time, the problems that arise can be addressed with solid advocacy, good communication, and practicality. Even more valuable are wisdom, kindness, and radical listening. While these aren't always readily on tap in a corporate setting, advocacy and strategy can help.

One of the first questions I ask a woman dealing with workplace related questions when she gets sick is the size of her employer. This is because the regulatory schemes that may affect a company vary according to the size of the company, and the ways a company makes choices is often dependent on the number of employees it has. For example, a company with seven hundred employees may have more flexibility in providing "reasonable accommodations" that may be required by law than a company with twenty employees. Most of the general legal requirements that become relevant when a woman gets sick apply to employers that are public and private, for-profit and nonprofit. It's usually just a question of the name of the law that applies. They may be federal laws or parallel state laws (which tend to apply to smaller entities). Not every version of these state laws are exactly the same, but most of the major principles are. I find it is helpful for a woman battling illness to understand the generalities of these laws but not to obsess much beyond that. An overview is useful not because most situations ramp up to a legal dispute (they don't), but because when communications and problem-solving commence, she will know where she stands and what she can expect.

The relevant laws that are engaged when an employed woman gets sick fall into the following big categories:

Antidiscrimination

Federal and state laws prohibit discrimination based on a person's disability and cancer, and most serious illnesses fit that bill. Under the federal laws called the Americans with Disabilities Act of 1990 (ADA) and the Americans with Disabilities Act Amendments Act of 2008 (ADAAA), employers cannot discriminate against qualified individuals with disabilities. Under the ADA, a *disability* is defined as a physical or mental impairment that substantially limits a major life activity. Most of the time, this includes cancer and other serious illness. Parallel laws apply to public employers, and different states have similar laws that apply to smaller employers within the state.

Antidiscrimination laws apply to all stages of the employment relationship, including hiring, job training, promotion, and termination. Here's what that looks like in terms of hard lines:

- An employer cannot transfer, lay off, demote, refuse to rehire, or promote an employee because that employee has or had cancer or a serious illness.
- Wages, conditions, and benefits for employees who have cancer or serious illness must be the same as similarly situated employees who do not have cancer or another serious illness.

- An employer cannot pass on to the employee any increased health insurance cost due to an employee's cancer or serious illness.
- It is unlawful to terminate an employee because that person has cancer or serious illness. Termination can be expressly stated by firing the employee or constructively demonstrated, as in a situation where the employee is "forced out" because the employer has made the employment situation untenable.

When I talk to a woman I'm trying to help, I keep it simple. The law prohibits certain behaviors on the part of employers, sure. But employers usually do what works for their business interests and find neutral ways to explain their choices, even this isn't entirely the case. Employment at will, a doctrine that posits that an employer can fire an employee for any reason in the absence of an agreement to the contrary, is the default standard in most states. Since few employees have employment contracts, what really matters is that a woman who is trying to keep her job and benefits makes all the right moves to achieve those results. It's not about setting up an employer for a lawsuit; it's about setting yourself up for security. The main idea I try to instill in the women I support is that their employer cannot take action against their interest *because* of their illness. As I mentioned in Stephanie's story, this isn't something to be used as a sword most often, but it can be a shield.

On-the-Job Accommodations

By law, an employer must accommodate a known disability for a qualified employee unless it would cause the employer an undue hardship. Generally, an employee must inform the employer of the disability when requesting a reasonable accommodation (unless the disability is obvious or already known to the employer). However, an exact diagnosis is not necessarily required if enough information can be shared with the employer to demonstrate a need for the reasonable accommodation. Doctors support these communications and help women with the right phrases to use to maintain as much privacy as they can while demonstrating the need convincingly. That's the big takeaway: ask your doctor for help. They do this every day and they know how.

As for the accommodations themselves, this sounds simple, but sometimes it can be hard to figure out. In a post-pandemic world, it is a lot harder for employers to claim that face time at the office is a hard-and-fast requirement, depending on the type of business. Accommodations might include scheduled breaks, backing out of certain tasks, job sharing, and time off for medical appointments. I encourage women to check out the Job Accommodation Network (https://askjan. org/), which is the definitive source of free, expert guidance on job accommodations and disability employment issues. In addition, I always urge women to suggest creative solutions that come to mind that may not be documented elsewhere. For example, a woman I worked with who was an editor simply asked her employer if she could work every day for two hours during her treatments. She liked having more flexibility and found that even on the weekends she wanted to be distracted from her illness. Just because something has never been done before does not mean an employer wouldn't consider trying it if it aligns with their larger goals. In fact, many employers appreciate employees who think about their employer's and team's circumstances and concerns.

Leaves of Absence

Employees who are battling illness are entitled to take leaves of absence from work to receive and recover from treatment. Federal and state laws, namely the Family Medical Leave Act and parallel state laws, lay out the rights of employees and responsibilities of employers in this kind of situation. Generally, these laws contain similar provisions, allowing for twelve weeks of unpaid leave during a twelve-month period for serious health conditions. These laws are the minimum standards that are required. Employers often choose to be more liberal because unpaid leave is a relatively inexpensive way to support an employee.

A key point for women who get sick is that employers must continue to provide health insurance for an employee on such a leave of absence, though no other employee benefits are required. At the end of a leave, an employee must be allowed to return to the same or equivalent job. If the same job is not available, the employee must be granted the same level of seniority, responsibility, pay, and benefits. Stephanie's time away had exceeded this twelve-week period, so her legal claim, if she'd made one, would have been regarding discrimination, not a violation of a "leave law."

When it comes to leaves of absence, a few things have come up that have surprised the women I've advocated for:

- Part of this leave period can be paid because of accrued sick days and vacation time.
- Some employers allow other employees to share or "pool" their sick days so that someone who is sick can use them.
- The leave does not have to be consecutive. It can be occasional or on a part-time basis to suit medical needs.
- After the twelve weeks have lapsed, an employee can request additional time off as a reasonable accommodation.
- While employer-provided health benefits are no longer required at this point, some choose to continue them in the interest of maintaining the relationship or as a statement of support.

Employee Benefits

Health Insurance

Health insurance is the most important employee benefit for employed women to consider when they get sick. It's the costliest and the most difficult to do without. Unlike retirement benefits or life insurance policies, which are future-looking, health insurance is a crucial, in-the-moment need. We'll talk more about how to keep health insurance once you have it in another chapter and how to get it if you don't, but here we will focus on the legal protections that a woman employee has once she is a participant in an employer-provided plan.

From a legal standpoint, it's simple: an employer cannot limit coverage, charge more premiums, or otherwise treat a woman differently when she is fighting a serious illness. But this does not stop employers from offering plans that limit certain coverage for procedures, treatments, and drugs. For example, many plans do not cover the caps that some women wear during chemotherapy to keep their hair from falling out. This is a newer device, and that's the main reason it hasn't been negotiated into plans, allowing insurers to say that these caps are not "reasonable and customary" and therefore not reimbursable. Over time, employers renegotiate their plans, but ultimately there's an appreciable lag time between medical innovations and their coverage.

Employers who make contracts with insurers are not breaking the law, nor are they ever required to offer richer plans. This illustrates why legal protections and benefits alone fall short when it comes to women getting the most humane, advanced care available. Often, newer devices, techniques and medications are out-of-pocket costs that women must either incur or avoid if they are prohibitive. This has the effect of highlighting the financial challenges already faced by lower-income women. Often, illness-specific support organizations will step in and facilitate the sharing and recycling of medical equipment and personal items like prosthetic wigs, caps, and other devices that may not be otherwise accessible to all. Workplaces sometimes refer women to these kinds of organizations, and some employers choose to support these organizations because their women employees turn to them.

While most of my energy is spent helping women keep their coverage, it is important to understand the basics of a health insurance plan. Covered items will vary from plan to plan. Plans that allow for out-of-network coverage often have complicated prequalification and reimbursement procedures. While some experimental treatment may be excluded, many states require health insurers to have an external, independent review process to review a plan's decisions regarding experimental or investigational drugs. If a procedure or therapy is viewed as historically unsuccessful or ineffectual, coverage will often be denied. In addition, anything that is not considered medically necessary may be excluded from coverage. Questions regarding whether an employee's treatments fall into any of these categories are complex, and answers can vary depending upon many factors. Employers can advocate on behalf of employees and often will. They are often better situated to know the details of the plans or at least the right contacts at the insurance companies to help employees get answers.

As I have often told women I support, employers are the parties to the contract with the insurance carrier. This gives them leverage that no individual employee has. When it comes to lining up a team to help support you when you need it, don't overlook the human resources department of your employer. One smart, compassionate person in HR can make a huge difference in your dealings with your health insurance provider.

Life Insurance
Some life insurance plans have waiver of premium provisions for individuals who are ill or disabled. This information should be outlined in the company plan booklet, policy, or Summary Plan Description (which is a fancy phrase for a plan overview that must be provided by law). If an employee's prognosis is poor, many life insurance plans have a *living benefit rider* that allows the individual to take out a significant portion of the life insurance benefit for current use. This amount, plus interest, is then deducted from the amount of the benefit paid to the beneficiary upon death of the insured. In some instances, employees use this money to fund experimental medical procedures that are not covered by insurance, but when a woman gets sick, that

is just one of the financial obligations she might face. Another thing I always explain to employed women is that if an employer provides life insurance and the policy has a waiver of premiums clause, that amounts to continued benefits at no cost.

Disability Coverage

Disability insurance is insurance that provides employees with some income (typically 50 percent to 70 percent of their salary) while they are unable to work because of a medical condition. Employees may have access to individual, employer-sponsored, and state or federal disability insurance programs. An individual plan is one that is purchased directly from an insurance company. An employer-sponsored plan is one that your employer provides as part of your employee benefits package. Both individual and employer-sponsored plans can be short-term (typically six months to one year) or long-term (typically longer than one year). Each type of disability insurance has a different definition of *disability*. Even when a woman has completed treatment, she may still experience side effects or have other medical conditions that keep her from being able to work. Most doctors have experience supporting disability claims, and it is always worthwhile to ask.

Additionally, employers will often support employees in the claim submission process. The process includes submission of medical information by doctors, as well as job-related information by the employer. Employees sometimes assume that the payment of disability benefits is solely contingent upon the opinion of the physician, but there's more to it. Of all the aspects of the employment and benefits relationship that I've helped women with over the years, disability is the most complex by far. It wasn't part of my original legal practice, and I've learned a lot along the way, but I almost always call in experts to help. Many law schools run free clinics that include labor law and disability sections. Experts guide law students in how to help clients, and I've sent many women to these centers to get wonderful help with disability coverage.

Pension Plans and Social Security
Pension plans sometimes provide additional income to women as they fight illness. Some plans have special disability provisions that allow for early or penalty-free distributions of plan balances. In addition, many plans have hardship distribution provisions and loan provisions that may help a woman who is facing a loss of income due to illness. Early retirement can be a viable option for some women when they get sick, whether it is under a private pension plan or social security. There are separate rules that are engaged in each case, but as I always tell women I work with, these are the benefits they have earned by working. They aren't charity.

Other Benefits to Look Out For
Many employers have flexible spending plans that allow employees to make pretax deferrals of income that can be used to reimburse employees for health-related expenses

not otherwise covered by health insurance plans. Anytime a woman must go out-of-pocket for anything related to her illness, these accounts can be used to cover expenses.

Larger companies have provided Employee Assistance Plans (EAPs) for decades. Generally, EAPs provide counseling referrals to covered employees, typically for a predetermined number of sessions with a mental health professional. Many women I have worked with have used this not-often-discussed benefit. With the rise of mental health awareness, an increasing number of smaller companies are providing this benefit as well. Traditional health insurance plans may also provide some coverage for counseling needed by employees, and this is another route a woman can pursue.

When I lived in Italy, I had many fascinating conversations that opened my eyes to the reality that the way we live in America is not the only way to live. We're obsessed with work here in the US. We allow our professions to define us and make assumptions about others based on theirs. Look at the average Instagram profile and survey the identifiers. There's always at least one that speaks to how someone earns a living. In Italy, I once asked a guy I met out for ice cream on the piazza what he did. He looked at me, perplexed, mirroring the question back, "What do I *do?*" I nodded as he rattled off a list: "I wake up, I have an *espresso* and a *cornetto*, I go to my office, I come to my mother's for lunch, I go back, and then I meet my friends for dinner. On the weekends, I go to the beach or sometimes the mountains." An *aha* moment.

His answer was fantastic. It showed me how narrowly I had thought about the question.

When a woman is focused on her health and healing, she may find a new perspective about just how much her professional life means in the grander scheme. However, I also believe that taking a hard look at what she's already earned by working, what her rights are, and how she can make sure to access the most support possible is key to an empowered health journey.

TIPS AND TAKEAWAYS

How long you have been at the company can matter for various reasons, but it primarily affects the possibility of early retirement, vesting in certain interests and possibly severance if a termination of employment appears to be on the horizon.

If you are employed and are currently on leave, a big question is whether your leave is paid or unpaid. In most cases employers will keep employees on group health insurance plans while they are on leave. Sometimes people will opt to be laid off, thinking that unemployment will be better income replacement than disability. Weigh this carefully, considering health insurance coverage, especially if you've had great or historically reliable coverage.

If your company has private disability insurance, ask an HR representative or a representative of the carrier to help you understand what you have. If there is none, you may be eligible for state or federal disability. Everyone pays into the social security disability system through their paychecks, but this system is extraordinarily complex. Get help from a dedicated organization on disability if you have questions.

Are other benefits available to you? Many people don't realize that they can take loans and hardship distributions from their own 401(k) plans without penalty. Other plans, such as employer-provided life insurance, may have cash value or other disability benefits. Uncovered medical expenses can also be reimbursed through flexible spending plans.

If you have a partner, it's important to ask your partner these questions as well, as clues to eligibility for some kinds of relief, or at least some understanding about the stability and availability of health insurance coverage, may be uncovered.

Try not to obsess about what's illegal. Think about what's practical. Do you really want that job anymore? Are you just in it for the income replacement and the insurance? If you do want it, stay in touch and interested even when you're "out."

Find out if your employer has joined the Working With Cancer Pledge (www.workingwithcancerpledge.com). This initiative, started in 2023, has changed corporate culture when it comes to cancer. Participating employers agree to:

- Provide salary and job security to workers battling cancer for at least one year.
- Offer career support to affected employees once they return.
- Provide custom support—including more flexibility— to employees who become caregivers to a family member with cancer.

{ 4 }

Taming the Health Insurance Beast

RECENTLY, I WORKED with a woman named Phyllis who was suffering with pain, nausea, weight loss, and fatigue and had been through a rigmarole of tests and appointments with various specialists. Understandably, she was anxious about her protracted journey toward a diagnosis. We talked about techniques for stress management, and I asked her if she'd considered therapy. She said that she could not imagine taking on another expense or making more phone calls or appointments. I understood completely. Her life was ruled by her MyChart, and she had grown accustomed to frustration. I asked her if she'd like some help researching what might be covered under her health insurance plan. To my mind, if she could find a helpful therapist, it would be a different and hopefully better experience than what she was going through. It turned out that there were in-network therapists in her plan who were taking new patients. The coverage wasn't indefinite, but it was great for the short run. Phyllis connected with a therapist who helped her more than she'd imagined possible. There are so many socio-emotional issues to contend with when facing illness, and what Phyllis was conditioned to perceive as another complication actually wound up helping her simplify and rightsize her feelings.

Do the Research, Get Advice

Often, women have better coverage than they think they have. It might take some research and effort to figure out what is covered, but when a woman faces illness, it can be worth her time. This is an excellent thing to hand off to a "chief of staff" and let her help you, because one thing is for certain: insurers do not chase women down to tell them about the benefits they're missing out on. Employers are not in the business of letting employees know the ins and outs of their health insurance plans. Even the best human resources departments put most of their energy and effort into finding comprehensive plans for their employees at different price points. Some may help employees troubleshoot when things go wrong, but few, if any, will proactively urge employees to take advantage of all aspects of the coverage. For these reasons, I always suggest that women take another look at their Summary Plan Descriptions, which are descriptions in plain English available for all health insurance plans.

It is hardly a revelation that the costs of health insurance and uncertainty around coverage are major stressors to Americans. At least two-thirds report cost as a significant worry.[1] Women and Latinx Americans are most affected by stress brought on because of rising costs and lack of access to healthcare. Fifty-seven percent of all "cost desperate" Americans, meaning people who say that healthcare costs are a daily source of stress, are women. Exacerbating an already untenable situation is the fact that 48 percent of all cost desperate Americans have three or more chronic conditions.[2] What this translates to is that large numbers of women who are unwell feel insecure about health expenses and health coverage. It is not an exaggeration to say that this has become both a cultural and economic beast. I have found as an advocate that the best way to help women think all of this through is methodically, because the complexity requires a step-by-step approach to analyzing available options.

Option 1: Seek Out or Keep Group Health Insurance

Group health insurance is always the starting point, because if a woman facing an illness has a group health insurance policy through her employer or a partner or spouse's employer, keeping it through a health journey is usually optimal. Staying on a group plan allows a woman to keep her doctors and manage expectations and stress effectively in most instances. She knows what the costs and patterns are and she will have less paperwork to worry about at a time when personal administrative tasks are at an all-time high. Group plans have more buying power with providers and increased leverage. Because they tend to have large numbers of members, group plans are less likely to be dropped by the hospital or healthcare system. For all of these reasons, I counsel women who are on a group plan to talk to human resources at their employers (or spouse or partner's employer) about staying on the plan for as long as possible through paid and unpaid leaves and disability periods. While no illness is stress free and no insurance coverage guarantees a perfectly smooth experience, I have seen many women's journeys on group health insurance go well with the right combination of forethought and advocacy.

Before the ACA was passed in 2008, people often were forced to extreme creative measures for staying on group plans, like finding a low-paying part-time job that hovered just over twenty hours a week during debilitating treatment. As I will go into at the end of this book, the rules that prohibit insurers from barring people from coverage because of preexisting conditions applied only to group insurance plans prior to the passage of the ACA, not individual ones, making individual ones nearly impossible to affordably procure after a diagnosis. In California, for example, the only way it worked for women I counseled was to go into a "waiting period" for a plan called MRMIP (Major Risk Medical Insurance Plan). This cost a fortune and delayed women from getting treatments they needed, adding appreciably to the already considerable stress of illness.

Since the passage and subsequent phase-in of the ACA, the biggest improvement has been more open access to coverage for people with preexisting conditions at the same prices that everyone else pays. Women may be less attached to staying on their group plans at all costs, though as mentioned, there are still reasons to try for that result.[3]

A few years ago, I worked with a woman named Charlotte who was on disability during a six-month cancer treatment. Her prognosis was good, but the medication she was taking made her feel quite ill, and her doctor supported her application to receive short-term disability benefits. Her employer's internal policy was to keep disabled employees on their health insurance plan for six months. Charlotte felt lucky that their policy lined up with her treatment timeline. Unfortunately, the company was struggling and began layoffs in her fourth month out. Employees in her group and her level, what we legally call "similarly situated" employees, were all affected, which meant that Charlotte likely had no claim for employment discrimination due to her disability, and she wasn't interested in spending her time suing her employer in any case. Charlotte wanted to keep her doctors, but she found herself unemployed and uninsured at the same moment. Normally, as I mentioned earlier in this chapter, I recommend extending group coverage, but in Charlotte's case, COBRA coverage was expensive enough that she decided to shop for a policy through her state ACA exchange. I was worried, but I understood the economic realities. COBRA coverage can be prohibitively expensive. I advised her to find out which individual plans her doctor would take, and she found one that was certainly not cheap, but it cost almost five hundred dollars a month less than her COBRA group plan.

It could have gone wrong. The doctors and medical system that Charlotte wanted to stay with could have dropped her new plan at the end of the year; this kind of shuffling happens often. Every year hospital systems and other medical providers audit the plans they contract with. If they've had a less than optimal reimbursement or preapproval experience, they may drop the plan. It's a numbers game, and if it turns out to be more trouble than it is worth and they believe they will have a steady flow of patients regardless, their incentive to continue working with a problem plan is low. Patients, unfortunately, may not know what is going on behind the curtain unless they ask.

Charlotte did her homework by making sure that her doctors felt that the carrier she bought the plan from was solid—that they regularly reimbursed for the claims they submitted, which decreased the chance that the medical system would phase out the contract. In an unexpected and interesting twist, they dropped the plan she would have stayed on had she paid more for COBRA, even though it was a group plan with many members. I was so happy Charlotte won this bet, though I wish women were not subject to this type of uncertainty. Choosing doctors should not be so fraught. Charlotte ended up with a better and more affordable outcome that let her stay with the doctors that she knew and trusted, but before the ACA was passed, this would have been a nightmare. Prior to the ACA, women with preexisting conditions of any kind were on a stressful course. Major risk pools, waiting periods, huge expenses, and a lot of uncertainty were typical. The situation is improved today, but there is still plenty to consider.

Another story hits home for me because it is about a close friend. After her divorce, she found herself in the unenviable position of having to find her own insurance, as often happens. Her ex-husband agreed to cover their three grown kids until age twenty-six (unless they got coverage through employment before that). At first, she stayed on COBRA to keep the excellent group coverage that her family had always been lucky enough to have. When she began to shop for plans, she saw that there was no individual plan available to her that could equal what she had. Additionally, one of her kids needed surgery and medications that would not be covered under his father's plan, and she wanted to support him as best she could. She realized she needed a comprehensive group plan to cover herself and her son and not end up paying exorbitant copayments and out-of-pocket minimums. She'd recently started her own business, an LLC, that hired some consultants, but not any full-time employees. All of them had insurance coverage from other sources. This seemed like good business, as she was running a small and tight ship and working toward profitability. But it turned out that she learned it was better to offer a group policy, even if her consultants declined the coverage, just to qualify for group insurance rates and better options for herself and her son.

All of this complexity and stress so she and her son could be treated by the doctors they each hoped to see. There was no other way to get this to work. Again, this is an example of divorce disrupting a woman's security and access to healthcare. It was a jump-through-hoops situation that shouldn't have been so complicated. But these situations often are.

I have seen people spend money to formally start businesses just to find ways to be covered under group insurance plans. This was more common before the ACA was passed because people with preexisting conditions could be excluded under by individual policies before it was passed. But even now, group health insurance is more affordable, comprehensive, and stable in terms of the contracts that carriers and employees are able to negotiate. In other words, group plans get dropped by medical systems less often because of the number of patients involved.

Option 2: Purchase an Individual Health Plan

When it comes to finding an individual insurance plan, the place to start is healthcare.gov, which will take you directly to your state marketplace, where you can find information about available plans, financial aid options, levels of coverage, and more. If you find it confusing or want to get advice, you can always enlist the help of a broker or go directly to insurance companies, but as a database, this is still the best place to begin to educate yourself. Women can take certain steps to optimize this process for themselves if they must shop for insurance mid-illness.

TIPS AND TAKEAWAYS

MAXIMIXING HEALTH COVERAGE

What is your plan, if you have one? The first step is understanding what your plan does and doesn't cover. For example, some newer procedures will be things you may have to fight for. Insurers are always slow to consider them "reasonable and customary."

Are the doctors you want to use in-network? This can make a huge difference depending on the terms of your plan.

Do you want or need second opinions? If you do, it can make sense to pay for doctors out-of-pocket, because money spent on someone's brains and experience, as opposed to devices, medications, and procedures, is money well spent. So, if a renowned expert in the field is not on your plan but you can get an appointment for a consult, take it and pay for it.

Do you know what your plans' copayments, deductibles, and caps are? This often trips people up. Copayments are cost-sharing for services. They are usually fixed. Deductibles are bigger sums that must be spent by the patient before full coverage kicks in and caps are large dollar figures that insurers will not reimburse beyond. In other words, they get you coming and going.

Have you checked to see if the specialists on your case—anesthesiologists, radiologists, et cetera—are covered to the same extent as your surgeon or oncologist? Remember to ask about all members of your care team, because otherwise you can end up with a bill you did not foresee.

Always call your insurance company with questions. If you do not understand your Explanation of Benefits, codes or words used, or bills sent.

Ask for and read the Summary Plan Description of your plan.

Use covered preventive services. They are usually no-cost and not subject to deductibles if they are in-network.

If you are worried about affording insurance or care, be proactive. Ask about payment plans, community resources such as disease-specific emergency funds, and premium assistance. Don't put off care or go uninsured.

Buying Your Own Policy

Think of health insurance as the key to opening the door to the care that you need, not a status symbol or measure of your self-worth.

Don't assume that the cheapest or most expensive option is best. Always match a plan to the doctors and healthcare systems you intend to interact with frequently.

Take a look at where you are in your treatment and health journey. If a clinic or an HMO has good facilities and personnel, and you are at the point in your treatment where important decisions about your care have already been made, you may find that a more modestly priced policy is a smart choice for you. If things change, you can always choose another plan at the next open enrollment period.

Here are the essentials to look for in every plan:

- Preventive and wellness services
- Chronic disease management
- Ambulatory or outpatient services
- Emergency services and hospitalization
- Laboratory services
- Pregnancy, maternity, and newborn care
- Mental health and substance abuse treatment
- Pediatric services, including pediatric dental and vision
- Prescription drugs, including brand name and generic medications
- Rehabilitative, habilitative services, and medical devices

You may want to consider a supplemental insurance policy to cover gaps or out-of-pocket costs if you anticipate travel expenses or high copayments.

Look into financial assistance for a state exchange/marketplace plan. Healthcare.gov provides premium estimates, and if your income is at or below 250 percent of the federal poverty level guidelines, you could qualify for reduced cost-sharing.

When you look at your coverage options in your state marketplace, consider your current medical needs and family medical history. Consider the following:

- How much would you spend on medications you are currently taking?
- What is your current household income? Are there any anticipated changes?
- How much can you afford to pay for out-of-pocket medical expenses?
- What are the deductible amounts that would need to be paid before your coverage kicks in?
- What is the plan's out-of-pocket maximum? After you reach your plan's established out-of-pocket maximum, every plan will pay 100 percent of the plan's negotiated amount for covered medical care.

Be careful with short term health insurance plans. They are not required to cover preexisting conditions. People think they are affordable temporary coverage. They can come in handy when someone is between jobs and the premiums are cheaper. However, some of these plans do not include prescription benefits, mental health services, preventive screening, or even hospitalization. Some states have limited the sales of these plans.

When you're choosing between marketplace plans, call and ask if your preferred providers are in-network and if your medicines are on the plan's formulary (the list of medications they cover). This information is not always up-to-date online.

Get help from an assister or a healthcare navigator for free. If you look at healthcare.gov/localhelp, you will find your way. These helpers are paid by the government to give you the information you need to make the best choices.

Stay away from unofficial, odd-looking websites and online ads. Scammers are looking to capture your data and sell you policies that may not be optimal or comprehensive.

Be mindful of deadlines and open enrollment periods. State marketplaces were designed to be easy to navigate, but there are bureaucratic hoops to jump through.

Know the difference between HMOs (Health Maintenance Organizations) and PPOs (Preferred Provided Organizations). HMOs have a tighter network of providers, and PPOs give you wider choices. That is why they tend to be more expensive. Know the rest of the lingo too: premiums, cost-sharing, deductibles. If ever you have a question, ask.

BASIC HEALTH INSURANCE TERMS

Authorization Approval from a health plan that is often required before receiving certain care, seeing specialists, or undergoing radiology scans or surgeries.

Claim
A request for payment for health services received.

Copayment and Coinsurance
Costs an insured party pays per doctor visit, in the form of a copayment (a fixed amount) or coinsurance (a percentage of the total cost).

Cost-sharing
The part of costs an insured party pays out-of-pocket. Cost-sharing usually includes deductibles, coinsurance, and copayments, not premiums or non-covered services.

Covered Benefit
A health service or item that is paid for partially or fully by a health insurance plan.

Deductible
The annual amount an insured party pays before the insurer pays for services.

Health Maintenance Organization (HMO)
Health maintenance organizations provide care through a network of doctors and hospitals. Care in-network is fully covered, sometimes with small copayments. When patients go out of network, they absorb all costs, except in some emergencies.

Preferred Provider Organization (PPO)
A PPO also has a network of providers, but if a patient elects to see out-of-network providers, your insurance will still cover some of the costs.

Premium
The premium is the amount a patient pays every month to be covered by a health plan.

In-network
Doctors, hospitals, pharmacies and other healthcare providers that have agreed to provide members of a certain insurance

plan with services and supplies at a negotiated price are "in-network."

Medicaid
Medicaid is a health insurance program for people with low incomes and people with certain disabilities. Medicaid is funded by both the federal and state governments but run by the states.

Medicare
A federally funded health insurance program for patients who are disabled or over age sixty-five. The original Medicare plan has two parts: Part A is hospital insurance with coverage including hospitalization, hospice, and skilled nursing facility services. Medicare Part B is medical insurance with coverage including physician services, medical supplies, and clinic care. Part C is Medicare Advantage and Part D is prescription drugs.

Medicare Advantage
Health plan options approved by Medicare and run by private companies. Often includes Medicare-covered healthcare, prescription drugs, and extras such as vision, hearing, dental, and health and wellness benefits.

Precertification
Approval from a health plan for an elective hospital stay.

Out-of-pocket maximum
The most an insured party must pay annually for covered health services. Once the out-of-pocket maximum is hit after

the deductible is paid, an insured party will have no more copayments or coinsurance and insurance will pay the entire cost of all covered health services for the rest of the year.

Referral

A referral is when a doctor sends a patient to another doctor for a specific, usually complex problem.

《 5 》

Even If You Have Insurance, Stay Prepared

HERE'S A STORY so dramatic my daughter thought it would make a good short film. And she's a filmmaker. My dear friend Maya had been divorced for about ten years. Her ex-husband, Michael, was diagnosed with a rare and terminal cancer. Even though the patient in this situation wasn't a woman, the people caring for him were *all* women: Maya and her remarkably smart, capable three grown daughters. Maya and Michael were on fine terms, though I wouldn't say they were close. However, when he became ill, she and her daughters rallied around him and made sure he was surrounded by his family during his last few years on earth. It was human and touching, beautiful and painful. One of the hidden gifts of terminal illness is how clarifying it can be. Conversations and acts of love are more openly approached when we know that days are numbered. When the journey was ending, the family was able to arrange around-the-clock hospice care for Michael in his home. The aim of hospice is humane: to keep patients comfortable. So many wonderful professionals work to make it that way for patients.

I remember getting a call from Maya one evening telling me that they believed the end was near. It was a tender time, and my friend was incredible about making sure Cynthia, the woman Michael was seeing was as much a part of the goodbye as she and her children were. She behaved like a gracious grown-up who understood that everyone was in pain. And they were, though they were laser focused on keeping Michael out of pain. I asked her if they needed anything over at his house, and she said that they were doing okay, all things considered.

The next day I got a frantic call from her.

"I don't know how this happened, but the morning hospice nurse is out of morphine."

"Isn't bringing enough morphine a *really* big part of that job?" I asked, incredulous and a little snarky.

"Yeah, I don't know. Listen, we called Michael's doctor, and they're phoning in the prescription to the Walgreens on University Avenue. Do you think you could run over and get it so none of us have to leave him?"

"Of course I can," I said.

I jumped in my car and waited in the line a few minutes, tapping my foot like the edgy New Yorker I sometimes am, before asking the people in front of me if I could please cut in front of them. They understood the dire situation and let me talk to the pharmacist. He spent some time scurrying about and searching his computer, eventually reporting to me that they did not have liquid morphine, only pills.

I tried to understand why they would not have called the doctor and told him that when they received the prescription, but realized quickly that I had no time to analyze the brokenness of the circumstances—all this tech and automation and here we are. People do what's in front of them. They don't look ahead and consider what might go wrong, and it is due to no moral failing on their part. The system isn't built that way, which is why it's crumbling from the weight of demand and inefficiency.

Back to the drama. I tried to keep my cool but pressed the pharmacist.

"Where can I get it quickly?" I asked.

The pharmacist said that he'd look it up, which took another few minutes. He named a store branch two towns over.

"Thank you," I chirped in a stressed way, "and can I ask you to transfer the prescription over there now and have them prepare it so I can hurry on to the freeway and deliver it? My friend is dying."

"Oh, no, you're going to have to get the doctor to call it in again over there, we can't transfer them," he said.

Unbelievable. I did some deep breathing. I knew better than to waste time arguing. There was no button he could push or call he could make. We were both stuck in a clown show.

I ran to my car and called Maya and reported this wrinkle. Enervated and grieving, she said she'd have her middle daughter, a skilled communicator with a business degree, call the doctor back while I sped down the freeway. I told her to make sure the doctor told them to have it ready. I got there about ten minutes later and did the whole "please can I go ahead of you; my friend is dying" thing again with the people in line. They were kind, as I find most people are. But I was losing my composure. Heart pounding, I told the fresh-faced pharmacist that I was there to pick up the liquid morphine for my friend in hospice that she was supposed to have waiting for me.

"Oh, I haven't had a chance to run the insurance yet. I can't pour the medication until I do that," she said.

"Listen, I apologize if I'm being pushy, but we are running out of time here. I need it now. My friend is in the end stages. I have to drive it over to his house, and it's fifteen minutes away. This is my second pharmacy, and the hospice nurse has no more. Can you please just pour it and run the insurance card afterward so I can get it to him? He has excellent coverage. I'm sure it will be no problem. His family is worried that he will die in pain."

"I'm sorry, but I can't do that. I'm not authorized. It's a controlled substance. There are rules I have to follow. Why don't you go buy some shampoo or something, and I will have it done in ten to fifteen minutes?"

Her hands were tied. I knew. But I persisted, asking if there was anyone else I could speak to. Baby-faced pharma-kid (I was beginning to feel ornery) said "nope." I was unraveling from the stress. I fumed, I paced, waiting to hear my name called. Instead, I got an awful text from Maya about ten minutes into my angry Walgreens death march.

"Don't worry about it," she said. "Go home. He's gone, and hopefully he did not feel pain, but we'll never know."

I'm not proud of how I talked to the pharmacist or how I harumphed around that drug store, but I also remain upset by what she said afterward.

I rushed the counter, pulse racing and blurted, "You know what? Forget it. He's freakin' dead." She looked at me with some empathy, but also confusion.

"What am I supposed to do now? I'm processing the claim! I'm not sure I know how to cancel it!"

"Not my problem," I said bitterly, my back already to her.

But you know what? It's *our* problem. All of us. Because this is insane. Good people, most of us. Role-players in this ridiculous push and pull. We all know this isn't working. Especially not for women.

Stay Detail-Oriented and Vigilant

As this story illustrates, insurance is the starting point, but not always the fairy-tale ending. While you may have paid an ungodly price, taken a job you didn't really want, or stayed in a union that wasn't working for you just to be covered, there may still be hills to climb. Be gentle with yourself and set your expectations. If you go in knowing it is unrealistic to expect everything to be plug-and-play, even though you have an insurance card with your name on it, you'll be less likely to be destabilized if something goes awry. The bureaucratic system, regrettably, is often stacked against the patient. It's designed to make claims and reimbursements arduous in order to reduce costs for insurers and purportedly patients, although that goal remains catastrophically unmet as healthcare costs remain astronomical. Still, if you anticipate some hassle, you'll be less shocked, and with the right support, things will work out. It's all about knowing who to turn to and what to do.

Ask Questions

Once you have tamed the initial insurance beast, there are pro-active steps worth taking to make sure that you apply the coverage you have to the care you need. Asking the right questions of doctors, health insurers, and medical systems in advance of treatments and setting up communication channels are the most effective things you can do to avoid bad surprises. Often something will not be covered that you might not expect, even if the doctor you're seeing is in-network for you. For example, if you need a procedure or surgery, there's no guarantee that every professional working on your case is also in-network. *Ask.* It could be that a medication prescribed is not covered. *Ask.* A choice about how to proceed may not be as neutral as it looks, depending upon the complexities of your coverage. *Ask.*

Your doctors may not be the people to ask, however. They've got enough to keep straight, and they are not typically the people working out the details with insurance providers. Also, changes happen all the time. There's a lot of cost cutting and jockeying that goes on behind the scenes. Talk with receptionists, schedulers, nurses, and nurse practitioners when you make your appointments and find out the basics of what might be covered based on your plan before you move forward with any treatment. They are the ones who know the latest, whether or not it's the greatest. Every time you move on to a new phase of treatment, you know what I'm going to say next. . . *Ask.* This can save you hours of Monday morning quarterbacking and poring over bills and forms. Even with all that italicized asking, there will still be things that you might not have anticipated, but you will be in the habit of questioning, ready to receive new information and react accordingly.

Rely on Someone

The way medical expenses are reimbursed (or not) by third-party payers is byzantine. Regardless of what kind of plan you have, I can promise you this: it's still going to be complicated, with questions at every turn, bills you may not have expected, and potholes you didn't see until they gave you a flat. Rather than internalize them, remain Zen and realize that where you start is often not how things conclude. It shouldn't be this way, but it is, so working on right-sizing your reactions to the twist and turns will serve you well. While I might not be proud of how I reacted in that pharmacy over the morphine delay, I certainly do not regret stepping in to carry some of that stress and frustration so that Maya and her daughters could focus on their final moments with Michael. So, I cannot stress this enough, *phone a friend.* This is the place to get help. Advocacy. Another brain on the problem. A voice on the other end of the phone. A patient person who can absorb some of the frustration for you, so you don't have to. As I've mentioned earlier, accepting this kind of help tends to be harder for women. Women are conditioned to be all things to all the people they love, to put a list of others first. There is no reason any woman should go through illness alone, and yet I'm sad to report that many still do, simply because they haven't imagined that there might be someone who would step up and help.

Anticipate the Complexity

It's worth getting into why things slip through the cracks even when a woman has health insurance. Most policies have deductibles, caps, copayments, rules for specialists, referrals, and the like. Specialists are siloed from one another, so not only do they not sit in the hospital cafeteria conferring about patients, they may not even know they are on the same team. They may not realize that they've recommended a course of action or a specialist that is not covered. Prescriptions are a whole other sphere, and controlled substances are tightly controlled, as you saw in the case of Michael. In the same medical system, one doctor can be in-network and another one out-of-network. Not only that, but in many cases, being underinsured can be financially less favorable than being uninsured. Sometimes, a woman can do better going to a county hospital where some care is subsidized than going out-of-network with a thin plan at an expensive provider. It could also be better to apply for a Medicaid plan if you're low-income, as opposed to struggling to pay for an inexpensive plan with minimal benefits. This can feel unclear. That's why every woman with a diagnosis or significant health challenge deserves advocacy. There's just too much dizzying information to assess that has nothing to do with healing itself. It's not a competence issue or even one of resources. It's a question of where to put your focus when you're wrestling with so much. I'm an advocate of advocacy for all women for this reason.

Pay Attention to Financial Matters

There's some good news in medical research, and many advances have been made with specific diseases. Of course, and my heart goes out to people who have lost loved ones to the cases we haven't cracked yet, and I know how that feels. I'm sad to say that in America there's hard news beyond the medical facts too: people end up in debt even when they are insured, and this often can be avoided with smart planning.

It starts with understanding that medications and treatments can be expensive, so many health plans require patients to pay thousands in the form of deductibles and other kinds of cost-sharing. Here's a sobering statistic: cancer patients are 71 percent more likely than others to have bills in collections and accounts closed for nonpayment. Here's another: two-thirds of Americans who have healthcare debt due to cancer in their households have had to cut spending on basics, including food and clothing. One-fourth have either lost their homes or declared bankruptcy. It isn't difficult to connect the dots further to see how this kind of stress can inhibit recovery and accelerate death. Researchers have already done that.[1]

A 2019 study showed that over half a million bankruptcies are filed because of medical debts, and the Affordable Care Act has not been successful in stemming this tide, particularly because it was under constant attack from 2016 to 2020. The goal of having more people insured was to avoid this or at least make inroads. Here's something people don't tell you—if you are trying to get a job, bankruptcy can make it harder. Many employers will move on from a candidate if a bankruptcy filing comes up in a background check—and they do surface, because court filings of that nature are a matter of public record.

Another problem inherent in the way the health space and the workplace interact is that the need for prolonged care can lead to job loss. That plus mounting medical bills can lead to homelessness as well as a lack of insurance.[2] The challenges compound. COBRA is a law that requires employers to offer former employees' coverage on their existing group plans for up to eighteen months (and in some states and unique cases involving disability even up to three years). But it isn't the employer or the government that pays the expensive premium, it's the individual, the former employee, or dependent, and it's expensive. You can see how this situation devolves quickly in many cases. In a recent conversation with a woman I know, I heard the way the COBRA decision panned out for her when she found herself between jobs and temping years ago, before the ACA had passed. It was all about the money. COBRA was too costly. She had to choose, instead, to skip her mammograms and wellness checkups for a few years because an individual policy was too hard to get because of her pre-diabetes and hypertension history. When her job ended years later due to the COVID-19 pandemic, she was at least able to find an individual plan in her state marketplace. The coverage was not as robust as COBRA would have been because the employer's group plan was more extensive, but she felt she had something to get her through anything catastrophic until she became Medicare eligible.

To add some vivid specifics, about one in six Americans has an unpaid medical bill outstanding, equaling somewhere around $81 billion of debt. Millennials, who also struggle under the yoke of student loans, rack up medical debt at staggering rates.[3] Having insurance coverage, by itself, is not protecting people from this.[4]

Having worked with many smart women facing cancer, I have come to understand why. This stuff is so overcomplicated that people on all sides have trouble finding the answers. The average patient will show up for treatments and appointments, pay their copayment, and expect that all is well. They don't dig into limitations and complicated authorizations. They just want to get care and get well. Who can blame them?

In June of 2022, the NPR column "Shots," which features excellent and in-depth medical news reporting, had a piece about people in America who are in medical debt. All the stories were distressing, but one really stuck with me: the story of Jeni Rae Peters. She is a single mom of two adopted kids and works as a mental health counselor. One of her children had been homeless. She also welcomes foster children into her home. In 2020, Peters was diagnosed with Stage 2 breast cancer. Today, that is a diagnosis that can be addressed successfully, but it often requires surgery, radiation, and chemotherapy. In her case, it did. Although she had insurance, Peters was left with more than $30,000 of debt. Bill collectors even showed up at the hospital when she awoke from her double mastectomy. She kept working to keep her insurance, even taking on extra shifts at the crisis center where she counsels teens, some of whom are suicidal. Some friends chipped in to help lower her debt. Still, her credit score cratered, and she worried about how she would care for her kids. In the article she talked about dropping her teenage daughter's car insurance and canceling ice skating for one of her foster children.

While Peters's cancer is under control and she's currently healthy, she's also continually threatened with legal action by debt collectors. She told the NPR reporter that she simply has no way to pay off what she owes. She's had bill collectors tell her it was her choice to get surgery.[5] She chose to live. That's the choice she made. This is not okay. It has never been okay. But injustice persists.

Some easy steps you can take are to never assume that everything is paid for, that billing departments are infallible or that your doctor's office has dotted every *i* and crossed every *t*. If you get a bill that doesn't make sense, call the carrier and be prepared to appeal. Reconcile yourself to the fact that it could take two rounds. Also not okay, but perhaps less devastating if you expect it. It isn't that any one person is a bad actor; it's that the system is so riddled with flaws, wrong incentives, bureaucracy, and regulation that it truly is a wonder that anything ever goes right.

Maya's ex-husband Michael was a man of means. He worked hard his entire career to have the status he enjoyed as a successful businessperson. He had the best insurance his company's money could buy and world-class doctors and treatments. With all of that, something as simple as making sure he had the appropriate pain medication when leaving this earth after a long cancer battle eluded him and his family.

I thought I'd seen it all, but that unattainable liquid morphine brought it home for me. The doctor sent in the prescription. He had no idea anything was wrong. The first pharmacist never told him that they did not have the drug, but the pharmacist was just doing his job, fielding the balls as they came at him. The second pharmacist was following protocol for controlled substances. Nobody was wrong, yet nothing went right. And this happens every single day in America.

Then there are those who are less fortunate. So often they are women, especially women of color. One unexpected bill can lead to a cascade of other challenges. One illness can change the trajectory of a woman's financial security and that of her children. It's a two-fold problem, one being getting through the maze and the other being not losing your shirt in the process. When it comes to cancer or another serious illness, there will always be another twist, with or without insurance. The system is that fraught. Just because you are covered or think you are doesn't mean there won't be an unexpected bill or an aggravating snafu, because the right hands and the left hands are not coordinating.

This is why every patient must self-advocate or bring a friend or professional advocate into the situation. Make lists of questions, bring legal pads, conduct follow-ups, use sticky notes, set reminder alarms on your phone—whatever works for you, but have a plan. This is the best way to save money and energy that should be harnessed for healing.

TIPS AND TAKEAWAYS

Once you've established your go-to team, sit down together and take a look at the basics of your plan: caps, deductibles, in- and out-of-network coverage, and systems in your area where you can be treated. This is table stakes before a woman embarks on a health journey.

Check with nurses, administrators, or physician's assistants at your doctor's office to make sure that the pharmacy of your choice actually stocks the medication you've been prescribed.

Make sure you and your home team know the names of the right people at your doctor's offices and inside the medical system where you get your care so you know whom to call or message to get answers when you need them. Pay attention to who answers messages in electronic portals, because often you'll find that these are the people with their fingers on the pulsebeat of the practice. They tend to know doctors' schedules and can often share your questions with them.

If your coverage is employer-provided, have the name of the human resources employee or representative at the provider who can help you get answers and maximize your coverage. People underestimate how much human resources professionals know about the ins and outs of the plans that their companies provide. Many of them know a lot.

Ask for a case manager at your insurance provider. If you're going through an illness, they will often assign one, but you have to ask. The benefit here is having a go-to person to turn to as opposed to a call-center person who is not familiar with your case. Every time you are connected to a call center, you're going to wait for the person on the other end to get up-to-speed on your situation. Sometimes you will get a person who is terrific and helpful, but that may not always happen. Case managers get familiar with who you are, what treatments you're having, and what your individual concerns are. They will often help navigate reimbursements and facilitate communication with providers.

❨ 6 ❩

Access to Advice, Diagnostics, and Treatment

THIS STORY IS about me. I'm high-risk for breast cancer. My mother was diagnosed at sixty and my sister when she was thirty-nine. Both have been through surgeries, chemotherapy, medication protocols, and as of this writing, neither has had a recurrence. My beloved maternal great-aunt Esther had breast cancer in her fifties or sixties. She had a mastectomy, no treatment beyond that, and lived well into her nineties. I was thirty-five when my sister was diagnosed a few years after my mother. All of a sudden, I was a walking statistic with two young daughters. Thus began my prevent-examine-test-biopsy-freakout journey. It's been over twenty years and, despite the anxiety, I know that I am one of the lucky ones. I have always had insurance and wonderful doctors who are supportive friends as well. But I have faced down layers of testing, waiting for biopsy results, and the stressors that come from doctors not always agreeing fully about what I should do next. I have scars on my body from a surgical breast biopsy and an ovary removal. Sometimes these imperfections bother me, but they also remind me daily how I have stayed on top of risk. Still, it's hard to be as vigilant as I mean to be without anxiety. Many women with my facts or similar ones choose more aggressive prophylactic surgeries, and I understand why: it clears the worry shelf. I have chosen a middle way of added breast examinations, frequent doctor's appointments, multi-modal imaging, surgery when there is something to remove, and more biopsies than the average person goes through in a lifetime. Part of my reasoning is that my mother and sister's cancers were not genetically similar, and we do not carry the BRCA-1 or BRCA-2 gene (though there are other high-risk genes), and some of it is that I have found a team of women doctors I trust, and they have guided me.

Even with luck and privilege, I have had challenges. When it comes to the question of how much screening to do, I have had a particularly angsty time of it. Specifically around breast MRIs. Generally, they are only approved for already diagnosed patients by most insurers because they are quite expensive. Certain patients who are high-risk can also be covered for breast MRIs, and there are a few tests that insurers use to figure out what constitutes high-risk. The more biopsies a person has, the closer they are to qualifying as high-risk, and while mine were all benign, I have had quite a few. After one over ten years ago, a trusted and lovely doctor who'd joined my care team to do one of my many biopsies pressed me: "Why aren't you having MRIs? Your insurance will pay for it!"

To which I replied, "But I hear there are so many false positives. I find all these biopsies scary and stressful. And I don't want to use more healthcare than I need just because it's covered."

To which my doctor replied, "I cannot understand why you wouldn't use a highly effective diagnostic tool that is available to you, given your risk profile."

I was stressed beyond words. I had fallen into a pattern of two physical exams a year with my surgeon, who had done the surgical biopsy for me when I was thirty-five. The procedure was basically a lumpectomy that took out calcifications that had formed on my right breast. When the results came back benign, my radiologist told me she had been pretty sure they were going to find a small tumor, which was why they had elected to take as much tissue as they took. Many days I felt strange and disfigured, so there was the extra emotional work of talking myself off that ledge. Plus, I was busy with the cycle. In addition to the bi-annual physical breast exams, I was doing mammograms and ultrasounds annually. I'd done genetic counseling and testing as well. On the heels of going through IVF to have my second child, I was tiring of being a perpetual patient.

When the question of adding MRIs into my mix came up, I called my surgeon for her advice, and she confirmed that there were a lot of false positives on MRIs because they pick up so much. She did note that it was true that sometimes early cancers were found, and of course early detection is key.

But she also told me that it wasn't clear that the outcomes of early MRI detections versus later detections through mammograms and ultrasounds varied at all. In other words, though MRIs picked up some cancers that mammograms and ultrasounds might initially miss, the time lag might not make any difference in terms of prognosis or treatment. But two other doctors I respected advised I should do the MRI. So I did it, and it scared the hell out of me. Though my results were normal and no-action-required, the experience, which I was not prepared for, was awful. I had not been told that it was a hospital gown, IV procedure. The nurses and techs told me they were happy to see me, and that I looked so great. They meant well, but they had never seen me before, and I took this to mean that they mistook me for someone who was a patient in active treatment. Between that and the "strip down, put on a gown" vulnerability, it set me off. An anxiety and survivor-guilt waterfall.

I talked at length with my surgeon about it. I told her how much I abhorred the experience. She soothed me and said I could choose to take a break. "Let's get you to menopause," she said. I was eager to hit that point because I knew that breast cancers were generally less aggressive for post-menopausal women. If I could get there, I thought, the terror would end. In the in-between, I had a scare with an ovarian cyst that looked messy on an ultrasound. I had the ovary in question removed by a doctor friend, the world's best and smartest ob-gyn. She removed my fallopian tubes as well, lowering my ovarian cancer risk, but she felt I should keep my other ovary and uterus for hormone health and total body well-being reasons. The nine days of waiting for the biopsy were excruciating, but after that, menopause came just a few years later, like a bittersweet blanket. In my head, lower risk for gynecological cancers was my new identifier. I swear it made me run faster. Perimenopause had been terrible, but once I crossed the finish line, I figured I was a whole lot closer to home free. If that meant night sweats, I felt that was no big deal.

The end of 2023 awoke me to the revelation that the journey wasn't over; I'd just entered a new phase. After years of my surgeon letting me know that my analytical and thorough radiologist always brought up the MRI, but that it was okay if I chose not to do it, something changed. I went for my mammogram and ultrasound as usual. My radiologist almost always asks for more images after the first few are taken, so I've learned not to flip out when it happens. But after all the testing was done this time, she called me into her office, as opposed to bringing me the "all clear" piece of paper and sending me off with a warm hug. This couldn't be good, I thought. We got through the pleasantries, and then she looked me straight in the eye, hand on her chin and gaze steely.

"Rebecca, I really can't understand how a smart person like you isn't doing MRIs. Your mammogram is fine, your ultrasound is fine. But I find early cancers on MRIs. The breast cancer rates are so high around here. And you are high-risk. I want to find it at stage zero or stage one!"

I was flabbergasted. Wasn't the real hope not to find it at all? That's how I was approaching it, but now I felt stupid. How could I, knowing what I knew, not be doing the right and best thing for myself when I could? When I fought so hard for other women to get the tests and procedures and treatment they needed? Was this the only way to look at it? From my doctor's chair, MRIs were the right and best thing. That much was clear. All those years I had no idea my radiologist felt so strongly. I thought she and my surgeon had an annual friendly chat and that all was well. I'm a lawyer. I even believed that doctors might put these things in files on purpose to show that they'd presented all options to patients. That made sense to me. It was the story I told myself and stuck with. But this intense conversation suggested a different narrative. It had been about ten years since I did the MRI and I told my radiologist what an emotionally trying experience it had been. I was trying to defend my past decisions and to let her know that this had a psychological element. We've known each other a long time and have always been friendly, but she was not budging.

"Every ten years is not going to be my recommendation. I'm not going to tell you I think this is smart. You can do this more often and you should."

I began to fall apart. Because this is hard stuff. This gray area where the patient is the one who makes the decision, filtering the opinions of different doctors. Even with all that I have seen and learned, I felt ill-equipped emotionally, intellectually, and spiritually. Usually, a good mammogram and ultrasound day was cause for celebration. But I felt deflated, scared and profoundly scarred. Sensing her frustration and disappointment, I told her I'd do it, that I hadn't realized she felt so strongly. But I walked home from the appointment in a tizzy. Later, I texted my surgeon and let her know how things had gone. She called me and we had a long talk. Her take was simple—she was neutral. She reiterated that the results, prognosis, and treatment if a breast cancer were found would likely come out the same whether we caught it earlier on an MRI or later on a mammogram or ultrasound. She said more recent studies confirmed this. But she also expressed a sentiment that I shared: she had known and respected my radiologist for years. She thought maybe we could put it off six months, since I'd just had a normal mammogram and ultrasound, but my radiologist, via text between them, pushed back, saying ten years between MRIs was too long and now was the time. My surgeon told me that if it wasn't covered, she wouldn't do it because of the expense. Again, a head-spinner. A week later I got a call from the imaging center and I reluctantly made the appointment, thinking if it weren't covered, I could wiggle out of the whole thing. Then I got the preapproval papers from my insurance company. I was back on the MRI horse, feeling jangled.

I dreaded the day, very early in January. What a way to start another year, I thought. I decided to at least be my own advocate. When I got to the facility, I had a brief talk with the woman at the desk as I was filling out my papers. I wanted confirmation that it would be fully covered. She told me it would be, all eye-popping $18,000 of it, except for the $300 toward my plan's out-of-pocket requirement that renewed in January (I subsequently got a bill for $970, which was not covered after all). I took the opportunity to let her know how hard it had been for me last time around. She was lovely and understanding.

"Look, really, this procedure is hardly ever covered unless you already have cancer," she said.

"I understand, and I know that being high-risk is an exception to that, but it's really unnerving to be treated like you're a 'regular' and with that distant, professional pity."

"Don't worry," she said. "We've got a great team back there."

The truth is, they *were* a great team. Professional, competent, and efficient. Perfectly kind in guiding me to my private chemo/IV room with the locker, sliding doors, and comfy chair. This time I knew what to expect. The scrubs, gown, and grippy socks were waiting for me. But even with the kindness and comfortable touches, I heard some things that convinced me that folks had been trained to say certain things, because I heard them ten years ago. Here are some of them:

"Are you here because something was flagged on your imaging?"

"I've seen you here before. You're looking really good."

"Every woman should get breast MRIs. They're just so
expensive that it isn't widely used for diagnostics."
"Once we get the results, we will make sure the doctors
do everything they can for you."
"I really hope you get better soon."
"Hoping for your cure!"

So kind yet so triggering. On the personal level, there I was
again, a patient caught in the matrix, feeling anxious and face-
less. My chart said I was there for prophylactic imaging, and I
made sure to emphasize it at the front desk, but every appointment is scheduled so tightly that there is no way each person
working on my case could take the time to learn that. So, I left
shaky and freaked out. On the larger level, my sense of justice
and fairness was engaged. If all women should get breast MRIs
and they don't because of cost concerns, this is yet another
example of the way our system prioritizes balance sheets over
women's bodies. Are the truths we are told filtered through the
profiteering of the companies collecting the premiums and
making the devices and drugs? It sure seems that way.

Analyze Your Options, Talk to Experts

My story shows that even with amazing insurance, fantastic
doctors who are genuinely concerned, and options for diagnostics, care, and treatment, anyone can be stymied and
stressed out by the system and its skewed incentives. In my

case, I had access; that wasn't the problem. It was the information flow and the lack of systemic clarity. When we allow third-party insurers to determine what is "reasonable and necessary," we've already given up the game. But this is how it works. The original idea that I should get a test because it was likely my insurance would pay for it, as opposed to whether it was actually the best practice, never sat right with me. The fact that there was an ongoing debate between doctors of distinction and excellent intentions exacerbated my discomfort. None of this makes sense. One doctor's idea of "gold standard" care may not even be available to most patients. And because women's health is less studied and lower priority, these problems continue to plague women.

The Fallout of the Long-Standing Lack of Medical Equity

Women work harder than men to receive advice, diagnoses, and treatments, even if they are well-insured. When they aren't, it only gets worse. And this problem is not even limited to the third-party payer system in the United States. In 2019, a widely cited Danish study out of the University of Copenhagen analyzing the data of nearly seven million people found that across various diseases, women are diagnosed later than men. The study looked at over 770 diseases and found that on average, women were diagnosed four years later than men. When it came to cancer, the gap was about 2.5 years, but in the world of metabolic diseases, it was an even longer 4.5 years. (The only exception was osteoporosis.[1]) If this happens in places where healthcare coverage is provided universally, imagine how the layer of struggling for coverage of tests, appointments with specialists, and the like might muddy the waters. Historically, women were not part of many of the medical studies that became the basis for widespread practice. It stands to reason that even for treatable diseases, the longer it takes to get a proper diagnosis, the further women are from treatments, cures, and management. How this lack of research disadvantages women will be specifically illustrated later in this chapter.

Digging deeper, women face more chronic pain than men, but are more likely to be written off as hysterical or hypersensitive. Dr. Elizabeth Comen's outstanding book, *All in Her Head: The Truth and Lies Early Medicine Taught Us about Women's Bodies and Why It Matters Today* expertly catalogs the history of women being misdiagnosed, maligned, and dismissed. It starts a crucial conversation about women's health. When helping clients I will often read the electronic after-appointment notes in their online charts. They are gratuitously referred to as *hysterical, anxious, reactive,* and *highly agitated* so often by non-mental health professionals whose job is to learn about their symptoms, order proper tests, and help them find a path to healing.

I've not seen a study on whether the incidence of this is higher for women than men, but I would bet that it is, and I can tell you that it does not promote wellness or make female patients feel supported, seen, understood, or heard. It makes them feel branded as "trouble" patients who will be locked out of being taken seriously when they are often desperate for diagnoses and treatment. Some of my doctor friends have told me that now they are afraid to write what they actually observe about patients' mental states because they can get backlash, which takes their energies in a nonproductive direction. Still, it seems women are singled out more than men, probably because of baked-in cultural bias. Beyond these notes, women are more likely to be told to their faces that the source of their pain is psychological. In general, women are prescribed less pain medication than men and more sedatives—there's your proof.[2]

According to researchers, these pervasive gender biases yield incorrect diagnoses and insufficient medical support. A category of disease that makes an excellent case study of the problem is autoimmune disease, because women make up 75 percent of people with autoimmune conditions. According to the American Autoimmune Related Diseases Association, a whopping 62 percent of people who suffer from these diseases have been labeled *chronic complainers* by medical professionals.[3] Then there's the heart disease question. While it remains the number one killer of women, their symptoms of nausea and fatigue, which are different from men's, are routinely branded *atypical*. But are they really atypical if we know what they are? Strain on women's hearts presents differently than it might for men. When it comes to heart disease, women are routinely undermedicated and undertreated, though these facts are known.[4] Given all these forces and layers, you can see why this book is called *When Women Get Sick*.

A Closer Look at the Barriers to Effective Diagnostics and Treatment

The barriers to diagnostics and treatment are more pronounced for women of color, under resourced women and anyone on Medicare or Medicaid. In chapter 2, I talked about my amazing friend Sarah. That story goes on because Sarah's multifactorial symptoms have continued to elude definitive diagnosis. Frustratingly, Sarah has been bouncing between specialists, always solving for who will take her Medicaid coverage and what tests will be covered. One of the reasons this is so difficult is that even within one medical system (and she has had to venture beyond one to get the care she needs), specialists do not coordinate, convene, communicate, and follow up. The most they do is read the records (which are now linked on Sarah's portal). One of the goals that Sarah and I have for the "next phase" is to get one specialist to talk to another one about her case. This sounds simple, but even with goodwill all around, we think it will take months, because getting messages answered, calls and appointments made, and anyone to step outside of the strictures of the system is that hard. It's been two long years. This is where strategizing and advocacy comes in, and I am determined to stay the course.

Access to Medications and the Lack
of Women-Focused Research

Access to medications is a whole other ball of wax. Because our system doesn't have single-payer bargaining power with Big Pharma, Americans pay more for name-brand drugs than citizens of countries with single-payer healthcare systems. Essentially, American consumers end up paying for the research and development costs, which get passed on. This has led to a rise in generics, which save third-party payers and consumers money but create their own set of problems—namely thin profit margins and intense competition and regulations that make these drugs a challenge to produce, which leads to shortages. Who does this hurt most? People with fewer resources, of course, as they are more focused on paying rent and bills and keeping food on the table, leaving them less bandwidth to advocate for what they need. They are also less likely to have flexible insurance policies that will pay for name-brand drugs. In December of 2023, Christina Jewett, an award-winning investigative journalist who covers FDA matters and other healthcare stories for the *New York Times*, wrote an article entitled "'I'm Scared to Death': Behind the Shortage Keeping Cancer Patients from Chemo." The article specifically highlights shortages in certain generic drugs, telling the story of a woman in Florida who was told she'd have to go forward with bone cancer treatment without two of the three drugs that were prescribed and proven to be effective.[5]

Her cancer spread, requiring amputations, outrage, and anxiety, not to mention outcries about how this could happen in such a wealthy nation. It stands to reason, as discussed earlier, that problems like these will disproportionately affect women.

Another way that women are not treated equally from a pharmaceutical standpoint can be traced back to research—or when it comes to women, a lack thereof. Dr. Lisa Cook, a leading internist who has worked with infectious diseases and was on the vanguard of the AIDS crisis, told me that she is not allowed to prescribe the PrEP (pre-exposure prophylaxis) drug for cisgender women that has proven safest for cardiac and bone health. She must use a drug that is inferior in this regard because the research has not been done on women, and the FDA will therefore not approve it.[6] I found this shocking, and apparently it is far from the only example. As we discussed it further, Dr. Cook pointed out the irony that women are more likely to face osteoporosis, so the fact that she could not give them the drug that was better for bone health was especially ludicrous.

How Laws Can Get in the Way of Protecting Women

Here's a story about how the laws meant to protect our privacy sometimes have a skewed effect and how access to information and treatment can be blocked. This story is heartbreaking, highlighting how our convoluted laws have had unintended consequences that hurt women. I met my friend Alisa Robinson Figueroa in New York City at a play about a high school women's basketball team contending with teen pregnancy among their ranks. It was a play full of themes, women's health among them. We got to talking, and Alisa told me that she lost a child, her beautiful daughter Diary Unspoken Truth. As happens when you meet someone you connect with immediately, Alisa and I wasted no time getting straight to the heart.

Alisa shared that her daughter had been born intersex and had suffered terribly from gender identity disorder and medical psychosis, as well as other physical health conditions, including heart and kidney disease, lupus, seizures, basal cancer, psoriasis, and female/male gynecological health issues. Her mental health issues were misdiagnosed, and she was often labeled as schizophrenic. It was a complicated medical puzzle. According to Alisa, medical professionals assumed she was transgender and decided to treat her constellation of symptoms with pain medication, leading to addiction. Diary struggled to get medical care, to be respected for who she actually was and to be heard. She wanted people to understand her origins and uniqueness, and she struggled to be recognized.

Diary bounced from rooms to shelters to cluster housing, including abandoned buildings with no security and limited lighting. Generally, these were places in high crime areas where members of the LGBTQIA community would be sent by the Housing and Redevelopment Authority. For a long stretch, Diary had refused living in more official facilities because she felt they weren't safe. Instead, she stayed on the streets or in drop-in shelters, at one point disappearing for three months. She subsequently escaped from a trap house in Brooklyn, where she was forced to use cocaine to dull the pain of being raped and abused. She was nearly murdered by strangulation because she no longer wanted to abide. During this time, Diary was in and out of hospitals and ERs all over New York but was never given long-term support or treatment despite her multiple diagnoses. Just prescriptions and discharges. As Alisa put it, "She would get diagnosed in the ER and then sent back out to live in the street. She was dying right in front of me."[7]

Alisa and her husband tried everything to help Diary. She was a legal adult, so they attempted guardianship, powers of attorney, healthcare proxies, and the like, but they found that the legal system and the healthcare system did not work together. It wasn't for lack of trying. Diary gave her mom important legal documents, including medical summaries, orders of protections, and a list of numbers and names in case something happened to her. But Diary was not well physically and mentally and therefore not able to cooperate with various bureaucratic demands, which is what it would have taken for Alisa to manage her care. Despite many years working in the court system herself, Alisa simply could not gain the power to act to help her daughter.

Then she hit the HIPAA Privacy Rule wall. HIPAA is a federal law and the Privacy Rule is meant to protect an individual's health information while still allowing health information to flow efficiently. It is supposed to protect the privacy of people who seek care and healing. People can waive this right, but they must be well and cognizant enough to do that. Diary was not well enough. This meant that Alisa and her husband could not access Diary's information and were never consulted regarding her care or told of her whereabouts or health events. Diary was smart and independent. She signed herself out of psych wards and pled her own case skillfully to reach whatever her goals were. Because she had a Medicaid plan, she'd often be discharged from hospitals after thirty days, when her coverage ran out, only to go to an ER and start all over again. She was falling between the cracks.

Alisa was facing what I call an imperfect storm. First there was the question of coverage, and Diary was not getting the care she needed because of the limits of her Medicaid plan. Next, it was impossible for her parents to act as her advocates and supporters because of the HIPAA Privacy Rule. Diary was in no condition to think rationally about waiving her HIPAA rights so that her parents could take an active role in her care. The person who gave birth to her and raised her, who, if Diary had still been underage, would have been her legal guardian, was locked out of the conversation, and it was harrowing.

According to Alisa, because of Diary's psychological challenges, many of her physical health issues went by the wayside. All the while, Alisa sought the help of aides, social workers, and homeless advocates. Tragically, nobody could move the needle. Diary was discriminated against for the way she looked, her drug dependency, and the struggles she was trying desperately to overcome, but it was a revolving door that ended in tragedy.

After much persistence, Diary's parents found an apartment for her, paying over a thousand dollars a month, but it was on a floor that had a lot of drug traffic, and it was clear that would not work for Diary. The family ended up using it for storage. Eventually, Alisa was able to find a place for Diary in a program through Housing Works in Brooklyn, a New York City nonprofit that fights AIDS and homelessness. This was after Alisa had been coordinating with her case worker for years. She knew it wasn't ideal and was known as "a bad environment where the crime rate is high in the area and lifespans are short." But it was worth a try and hopefully safer than the street. Diary had been having frequent seizures when Alisa got the call for the apartment. Her last words to Diary prior to accepting the place were "I don't want to find you dead on the streets."

Diary was relieved to have a place to stay. She brought Alisa the key to the place to show her, and mother and daughter felt glory and comfort. In the two weeks she lived there, the people at the shelter grew to know her and love her. But Diary was unwell and still not consistently getting many of the medical treatments she needed.

Diary called her mom on a Thursday, and Alisa knew as soon as she heard her voice, saying "Mommy, I'm feeling very sick," that it would be the last words her child would speak to her. Choked up, Alisa told her, "I am preparing some clothes for you," because Diary seemed to keep losing her things. By Friday, Alisa had a sinking feeling. She'd hoped that they'd be doing wellness checks at the shelter, but she knew from trying before that if she called, she would get no answers. HIPAA blocked the release of any medical information. The weekend came and went.

Because Diary was afraid for her safety and had been raped before, she tried to tie up her door. There was only one lock, so she added a chain on the knob for extra protection. On Monday, Alisa got a call from police officers reporting that Diary had been found dead in her closet. At first Alisa worried that she had been murdered, but upon speaking with the officers, listening to the media, and scrolling through Facebook, she was not convinced. Alisa coordinated with the coroner because Diary's body had already decomposed, and the coroner explained that a traditional autopsy would not be possible. In the meantime, the media and LGBTQIA community got involved. Headlines talked about the death of a trans woman. Social media took it to another level. Alisa was unable to delete Diary's profile and almost got hacked in the process. The coroner advised Alisa that a bottle of seizure medicine was near the body, and it was possible Diary died of a seizure and was fighting for dear life to save herself, but this never made the news. As her mom states, "My child became a statistic, but not on the streets." In that respect, if not others, Alisa's prayers were answered. Diary had a roof over her head.

Alisa prepared an obituary for Diary, including a "Last Will," which Alisa wrote in Diary's voice. With her permission, it appears below:

LAST WILL

written by: Alisa Figueroa (Mom)

I have no material items to leave behind, I have my great smile, laugh and legendary personality to remember me by. I am tired now. Constantly always on the go, only my loved ones know. I will leave you by saying I did show the world I was the scars and beauty of Diary Unspoken Truth. It's my everlasting nap time now. My early calling is over now. I'm at peace and rest now. My spirit and unspoken truth will live on through the memories of my loved ones.

At Diary's memorial service, Alisa spoke with the CEO of Housing Works, who told her that since many of the organization's clients/tenants are dying anyway, the HIPAA Privacy Rule was often invoked to let them do anything they wanted behind closed doors without any reporting or monitoring. Alisa is haunted by the lack of information and the way the complicated, layered social service and legal system failed her daughter. To fill Dairy's void and help others, she advocates for revisions of the HIPAA Laws. If HIPAA had an exception for next of kin to be given access to medical information in extreme situations like drug addiction, psychological distress, and homelessness this could have gone differently. Alisa hopes that HIPAA can be amended to realistically consider the psychological issues that legal adults are contending with so that loved ones can be more involved in their care. She hopes for a day when there is recognition that there can be physical and medical issues intertwined with psychological struggles that should not be used as a shield to keep out help by the people administering healthcare services. Alisa believes that the LGBTQIA community faces widespread discrimination and that legal carve outs designed specifically to protect them and give them streamlined access to support and help are in order. As she puts it, "A lot of these kids are on the street already, and when people live on the street and are abused and taken advantage of, it's an ongoing cycle. We cannot let those who run transitional housing for the homeless with medical issues and addictions use the HIPAA laws to let their tenants/clients do anything that want behind closed doors while shutting out families and loved ones." Alisa is still walking in Diary's shoes for justice, and Diary still lives through her.

Alisa and I have become good friends. We can imagine fixes to a problem like the HIPAA barrier she faced in getting the best care for Diary. Though the law was designed to protect patient privacy, it was an unquestionable barrier for getting Diary the diagnostics and treatment she needed. It cut her parents off from information about her condition that they could have used to effectively intervene and advocate for her. As Alisa and I have discussed, problems like these require methodical action.

The first step is telling the stories and raising awareness about the ways that a law like HIPAA can block a woman on a health journey from accessing the help she needs. These stories are complicated and take time to unfold; they are not neat sound bites. It is my honor to tell Diary's here. The next steps are smart coordination resulting in legislative changes. For so many women, bureaucracy is getting in the way. Setbacks like a lack of research, corporate greed, and laws written without deep understanding of what real people face and systemic discrimination lead to more challenges. Health and social services do not coordinate, and this can keep women from accessing care and community. We have to do better by untangling this. Patient by patient. Woman by woman.

TIPS AND TAKEAWAYS

Every woman, regardless of her coverage or condition, can benefit from a thoughtful review of her options and advocacy when considering access to advice, diagnostics, and treatment. There will always be more to a situation than meets the eye.

It's always worth doing the research about the kinds of tests that are "normal" for what you may be contending with, but keep an open mind when you talk to your doctor. There may be complicated concerns about cost, coverage, incidence of false positives, or risks that outweigh benefits. Always have testing on your list of questions and listen carefully to the answers. Sometimes you will need to advocate for a procedure or a test, other times you will be offered options. All of this can be confusing in its own way, so the best course is to get more than one opinion and consult your support team if you feel overwhelmed.

On the topic of researching a condition, be careful with the Internet. Even when the source is reputable, statistics can be misleading. The Internet knows a lot, but it doesn't know you. Steer away from jargon and journals, because the specialized language can throw you off or send you down a rabbit hole. Your doctor and other medical professionals should always be consulted because they have experience evaluating the facts, studies, and circumstances.

Medical trials are happening all over the country for many conditions. Ask your doctors about the right databases to check, and see if they know of any studies that you might be a good fit for. When looking into trials you'll want to learn about side effects, the experiences of participants, and the credentials of the doctors running the study and phase. For many women, trials can be a way to receive lower cost or free treatment in a controlled environment.

Your specialists and primary care doctors may not communicate much with one another unless you ask them to do so. Often nowadays, they will rely on centralized electronic medical records. Be an active participant in your journey and encourage collaboration when you think it is needed. In some cases you may be able to message them in a group through your patient portal.

If you want to bring your advocate or another member of your team to any appointments, make sure to let your doctors know you prefer this and that you are willing to sign any necessary waivers.

〔 7 〕

Communicating with Your Doctors

BUILDING ON THE personal stories I shared in the previous chapter, I begin this one with a story about a doctor I've already mentioned, my breast surgeon. She's been on the front lines with me, helping me to manage my high risk for breast cancer. It all started with calcifications on a baseline mammogram that I had at the age of thirty-five, which I shared about in the previous chapter. The normal, insurance-approved age to start mammograms is currently forty, but I had that screening done early because of my family history, and that is why insurance approved the scan. While so many strides have been made in the fight against breast cancer, one alarming trend is the recent rise of diagnoses among younger women.[1] This may eventually result in earlier screening protocols across the board. When I was thirty-five and having this baseline mammogram, I had two small daughters, seven and three. As part of that first time, my radiologist (the same one I talked about in the previous chapter) asked to repeat a few angles. Not the kind of callback anybody wants to get (though as I mentioned, I have grown accustomed to them). After the imaging I sat down across the desk from her, heart beating fast, mouth dry. She told me she saw calcifications on my right breast. I had no idea what that meant at the time, but I could tell from the way she was talking that she suspected something, and she referred me immediately to a surgeon she worked with frequently. I will never forget our first phone call.

"Hello, Rebecca. I looked at your films and I want to tell you that whatever you've got there, it's very likely to be small, and I'm going to get it out."

This communication gave me confidence and hope when I was too emotionally paralyzed to access either. It was all about the way my wonderful surgeon talked to me. A seasoned professional, she knew the territory and blended her experience and compassion to choose the right words at the right time. She never said "I guarantee you, you don't have cancer," or "I will not let you die." Of course, that is what I wanted to hear, but no doctor can say this. The words she chose were enough to calm me and help me face whatever was to come. That's a neat trick.

Doctors Deal with Unseen Challenges

I've had the privilege to know many doctors. Close friends and family who have pursued the years of education and training it takes to put on a white coat and treat patients—it's a long slog and the conditions have changed, with escalating costs and increased business management. Many of my friends and the physicians I am treated by no longer transact with third-party payers; they just provide the receipts for their patients to submit to insurance on their own. The story is always a variation on this theme: they want to practice medicine, not be paper pushers; they want to take care of patients, not negotiate endlessly with insurance companies. From the outside they catch criticism because it puts more responsibility back on patients, but for many it's a combination of survival, burnout avoidance, and frustration from years of wrangling to get treatments covered for their patients. Other excellent doctors have joined large systems or HMOs so they can practice with the backup of an organization that will do the administrative work. There are trade-offs, like tight windows for seeing patients, strict rules for how and when to record patient information, and weighing costs as part of treatment decisions. Quite a few doctors I know have resigned, retired early, or joined concierge practices, which are a different model entirely. A concierge practice is where, for a large fee, people can reach their doctors immediately, be seen quickly, and skip a lot of red tape. Of course, this kind of care isn't accessible to most people, and for some doctors it is a difficult decision to make because it cuts them off from all but the most privileged of the patient pool.

The United States has a massive shortage of primary care physicians, and not only in remote areas. Doctors are worn down, especially primary care physicians, who are expected to quarterback patient care with specialists. According to the Association of American Medical Colleges, the US faces a projected doctor shortage of between 37,800 to 124,000 physicians by 2034.[2] This is despite a rise in medical school enrollments. Medical schools aren't keeping up with population increases, and a growing percentage of medical students skip the system and patient care altogether, going into biotech and medical venture capital. Another challenge is that there is a residency shortage, another roadblock to doctors practicing.[3] As with other stresses on the system, it is the underserved who are impacted most.

Ask Yourself What Kind of Relationship You Want with Your Doctors

In approaching the doctor-patient relationship, I counsel women to consider what they're after. Finding the right doctors is a layered process. I ask women to ask themselves: Do they want the most seasoned person, the doctor with the highest ratings, a person who will spend the time to talk things over, or something else?

The best a woman can do when she's on a health journey is start from what she wants in a relationship with her doctors. Dr. Kristina Austin, an experienced ophthalmologist, did a highly articulate job of laying out what this can look like when I asked her:

There are certain patients that may not do well with me, they may want a dominant male to be telling them what to do. I like to engage the patient

in a mission we're on together because I want them
to change a behavior or create a new habit, and I
have to have them buy in with me that they know
why I'm saying it. Not everyone wants that kind of
partnership with their physician. Some just want the
white coat, made decision and not really explaining
too much. People do better with different personalities
and we're all different.[4]

Dr. Austin's point is well-taken. They say expectations affect how we feel about our experience, and while I've never been quite sure who "they" are, I think they're right. I always recommend initial consultations with more than one provider because even with proactive expectation setting, comfort and instinct play a role too. A woman might find that the best "on paper" doctor is not the one she feels most at ease with. Though it takes effort and some extra phone calls, it is worth it to talk to more than one doctor before embarking on a health journey.

Consider How You Communicate with Your Doctors

Once a woman has chosen the doctors that suit her preferences, assuming she has a choice (given the vagaries of insurance coverage and wait times for appointments, this will not always be the case, and it can be a labyrinthian exercise), the next thing to consider is how to communicate well. This is a two-way street, and while it isn't always easy to keep anxiety in check and be a patient patient, being respectful and clear is the place to start.

Doctors are human beings. People who have chosen to devote time and effort to learning how to help heal others. As a lawyer, I've noted that doctors and lawyers are often grouped together, a kind of vaunted, well-paid professional trope, but also the recipients of a heap of generalized criticism. Short-hand monikers are full of negative associations (such as *lawyers are argumentative and bill-driven, doctors are dismissive and ego-driven*), but behind the curtain, doctors and lawyers are people who want what most of us want, to use their gifts and be respected. I've often thought about how many problems we could avoid as a society if we were to stop treating people as categories and start treating them like individuals with beating hearts and independent minds.

The way patients and doctors communicate can make such a difference. Whenever I advocate for a woman inside of this system, I remind her of this from the get-go. Doctors are not gods. They are educated, experienced, and worthy of deep regard. They have human needs and feelings, too, and they are under stresses of their own. I had an illuminating and specific conversation on this topic with Dr. Amanda Hoover, a board-certified internal medicine physician with more than twenty-five years of direct patient care experience, author of two books about patient empowerment, and founder of a curated education site where people can learn valuable information about how to maximize health and wellness. Dr. Hoover mentioned that mutual respect is the key. As she put it, "There may be times that the doctor's overbooked and you want to be seen. Nobody in the world could blame the doctor for not working you in because she is already overbooked, but maybe if that doctor has a very high opinion of you, maybe she's going to work that extra half an hour instead of going to her kid's softball game, and bring you in where she is not obligated to do so." Dr. Hoover told me that finding common ground helps in cultivating quality doctor-patient communication. "If there is an opening to mention something that will bring you guys together like, 'Hey, I bought my husband some boots like that,' that may break down some boundaries and make the doctor smile and say something like, 'I got these on sale. I have three pairs like these.'" Personalizing the interaction helps gives doctors a way to connect. Dr. Hoover elaborated, "When a doctor develops a relationship with a patient that goes beyond, 'This is Mrs. Jones, this is a disease called diabetes,' to, 'This is Mrs. Jones. We both like the same things. I can't wait to see her today,' that's what you want."[5]

For optimal communication, setting parameters is crucial. Be clear and ask your doctor how she prefers you to reach out when you have questions. Find out her availability, how she likes to be contacted, and what you can expect in terms of response time. Doing this in advance saves angst and creates space for respectful exchanges and fewer misunderstandings.

Part of being thorough and thoughtful is finding out who the go-to person in each doctor's office is for your questions. For example, doctors usually aren't the ones to ask about coverage or scheduling, but office administrators are typically well-versed in these topics.[6] If it's a question of drug dosage or treatment protocol, that is likely to be a question for the doctor. When you respect and get to know the nurses and administrators in your doctor's office, an added benefit is that they will advocate on your behalf and get messages back to the doctor for you. Nurses are amazing sources of information. They know about medications, side effects, devices, and practical ways to address problems like swelling, unexpected pain, and other complications that may arise.

Dr. Austin told me a story that illustrated a version of this point but also showed how things do not always go according to plan and can get messy. She was trying to make an appointment for herself by phone and was put on hold and eventually told that her request would be referred to two clinics where she hoped to be seen. One never called her back, and she missed the return call from the other and could not get back in touch. If you've tried to make appointments with a large medical system, none of this should sound foreign to you, but Dr. Austin was a senior doctor *inside* the system and still could not connect. So, she did something that she knew was ridiculous but that she also believed would work. She emailed her doctor apologetically, saying, "I'm so sorry, please forward this to your medical assistant to make an appointment for me.

I really need the treatment, thank you."[7] She got the appointment but continues to reflect on the absurdity of having to bother the very person that the layers of administrative support were meant to insulate from these kinds of tasks so that he could practice medicine.

In chapter 6, when talking about how research can affect women's access to medication, I mentioned Dr. Lisa Cook, an internist with years of experience treating infectious diseases. Not every doctor will be as expansive in her thinking when it comes to patient care and communication as Dr. Cook, but her attitude can be an example for every stakeholder in a health journey. When I asked Dr. Cook how she handles this first step in patient-doctor communication, she said, "I just give them my cell phone. Because it's better to communicate directly and hop on a call and talk when we can. I ask them to tell me how they would like it to go. Would they like me to call them once a week at a specific time?"[8]

I asked the obvious question, whether she was worried that people would take advantage of having her personal phone number.

She didn't hesitate. "Listen," she said, echoing Dr. Austin, "I've been a patient too. We are all having to deal with voicemails, electronic health records, and portal messaging. It isn't working. I have seen if for myself. My patients end up respecting me because I respect them."

There it is. She treats her patients like people, and they feel confident and seen. They don't escalate non-emergencies or act out of anxiousness because Dr. Cook makes them feel calm and cared for. While I know that not all doctors are as clear-eyed on this subject or as generous, the principle is there—setting respectful expectations in all directions goes a long way.

The Role of Electronic Health Records

An analysis of the role of electronic health records and portal messaging is warranted, as it occupies such a large place in patient-doctor communication nowadays. Not all doctors feel the same way about these systems, and they are typically chosen by businesspeople who work at the provider and are marketed heavily by the companies that conceived them. While they have improved access to information for patients, they have created many challenges as well. Patients often feel cut off, treated like numbers, confused by what they read or by the complexity of these portals altogether. Some doctors find these systems troublesome too. As mentioned in chapter 6, doctors do not always feel at liberty to write freely about their observations. Dr. Cook pointed out that another chilling effect of doctor communication extending from the "patient as audience" development is that patients will rate their doctors and their experiences with the medical system. Dr. Austin has similar thoughts. According to her, doctors censor themselves to avoid negativity. She relates that in the past, she might have said that it was difficult to pinpoint a patient's history and that perhaps the patient was vague or rambling. "I can't write that now," she says, though it might have been useful to have in the records.[9] It's part of the way medical care is marketed, managed, and monetized, the feedback loop. You might call it the YELP effect," or as Dr. Cook says, "as though your experience with a doctor is akin to a hotel stay."[10]

And that's not all. As she notes, these systems were originally meant to make communications among teams and specialists more streamlined (and that is the best use of them, according to Drs. Cook and Austin), but they have become places where patients read test results and reports before their doctors do, creating anxiety, alienation, and search-fatigue for patients. Quite often, words like *mass, irregular, abnormal,* or even *unremarkable* will send a patient on an Internet chase that stokes fear and confusion. This could easily be avoided by a conversation with a doctor. However, once a report is posted, often a patient will read it without guidance. Dr. Austin believes patients should not read physician's notes either. She feels that most don't know how to interpret the jargon and will use lay assumptions for words in a medical context, causing them often to catastrophize or misunderstand.

Electronic health record systems also make work for overburdened doctors who already have so much going on behind the curtain. Dr. Austin reports that filling out forms and checking boxes is something doctors are asked to do while seeing patients in limited windows. Instead of talking face-to-face, they are often meeting patients with eyes and hands on computers or tablets. This stymies the up-close communication and examination that patients want from their doctors, which many doctors strive earnestly to give to their patients. As Dr. Cook explains, there are other forces at work. "Everything's been bloated with administrators and financial people salivating over the electronic health record. Once we got them, the meetings went from 'let's discuss cryptococcal antigen and the fungal infection of the brain and this kind of small cell lung cancer' to 'how do they want you to tweak your note to make sure it will be inoffensive and potentially a way for the medical system to recover more insurance reimbursement?'" Dr. Cook told me that protocols for asking questions of patients have been developed specifically to allow a system to code and bill at a higher level. For example, in a straightforward appointment for a set of physical symptoms, if a doctor asks two more questions about social history and one more about family history, the appointment can be billed and coded at a higher rate, as though more care is being given. It could be largely irrelevant to the patient or the care. But it happens because the incentives are to recover as much money for each doctor-patient interaction as possible. Dr. Cook acknowledges that the horse it out of the barn when it comes to electronic health records, yet she hopes that the system can change again because as she puts it, "suddenly billing and coding and documentation took precedence over patient care."

Another important topic in doctor–patient communications is precision. To drive toward the best outcomes, it makes sense for patients to prepare in a two-fold way. The first is to come with specific questions written down, because it is common to freeze up with anxiety or go out-of-body when you finally get to see your doctor. For women, the added "go along to get along" tendency that so many societal forces have created is a challenge. The fix is to have the questions and concerns pre-articulated; it makes the act of asking less of an effort. It's okay to read them like a script, whatever it takes to get the information you need in the limited time you may have with your doctor.

Be Specific About Your Symptoms and Circumstances

A second aspect of tailoring the way you communicate to the best effect is in the descriptions you use when telling your doctor about the symptoms and side effects that you're experiencing. If there are details that you think will be relevant to actions your doctor suggests, try to make them as clear and accurate as possible. For example, rather than talking about stomach pain, if you could guide your doctor more specifically, say, to the left upper quadrant of your abdominal area, that might provide your doctor with more useful information. Dr. Hoover helped me understand another aspect of how delivering information to your doctor can help you get what you need. She told me a story about a patient who told her, "Doc, I can buy my medicine or I can eat."[11] Dr. Hoover put it like this:

*You have to meet people where they are. You can use
all the fancy, new fungal drugs in the world, prescribe
all these things, and if they can't get it, what's the
point? If you know that this person is on Medicare
or Medicaid and those plans are not going to cover
something, or the person is unemployed and you can
get a four-dollar prescription for this person, it may
not be as good as the brand new medication, but it
can keep the person out of the ER and keep the person
from having a massive stroke. So, I want to know
what's realistic. You need to know what the person
can afford. Just ask people. I'm not trying to pry in
your business, but I need to know what's realistic.
Is fifty dollars a month too much for you for a
prescription? If the answer is "Yes, it's too much," then
that door is closed. I'm not going to use that drug. I'm
going to use another medicine the person can afford.
There are other realities too. Can I get somebody to
take me to the other side of town to see this doctor,
realizing I can't drive and my kids live out of town
and I can't take a bus because I'm disabled? You have
to look at the whole patient; otherwise, you're really
not doing the person any good. The more prepared
a person is before he or she walks into the doctor's
office, the better that person will be prepared to tell
the doctor what's likely going on, and the doctor can
narrow down the diagnostic possibilities and focus on
what's important.*

Being open with your doctor about what is possible for you and the parameters of the challenges you may be facing will go far. As discussed earlier, women are culturally conditioned not to ask for too much and may feel shame or discomfort in letting a doctor know about financial or logistic concerns. Most doctors, however, will appreciate having the complete picture.

Women's Pain and the Hysteria Myth

There are myriad studies to back up the assertion that women's pain gets dismissed or ignored—it is a matter of so-called epistemic justice, because women's credibility is called into question on a systemic level.[12] Historically, women have been branded *hysterical* by our medical system. As Dr. Hoover says, "There has traditionally been a disparity in healthcare. Women's symptoms are often considered to be due to their anxiety, and men's symptoms are taken more seriously. That is an area of significant concern because I think a lot of diagnoses have been missed and the appropriate care was not rendered, assuming that the woman was just being hysterical. Well, of course, if you're having chest pain from a heart attack, you're anxious. Men, they express themselves differently. Sometimes women's symptom shifts are not taken seriously, and so the medical profession needs to do better at treating women with the same level of caution as they treat men and not brush off their complaints as something that anatomically doesn't fit the textbook, or whatever the case may be. We have a ways to go with that." Indeed.

To crystallize the problem, one need look no further than the award-winning, widely downloaded podcast, *The Retrievals*.[13] Hosted by Susan Burton, the podcast tells the stories of women who were reproductive endocrinology patients at Yale New Haven Hospital in 2020. A nurse assigned to their egg retrieval procedures swapped saline in for the fentanyl to be used to alleviate the patients' pain. Women were routinely manipulated and gaslighted into the belief that the extreme pain they expressed was either normal or exaggerated. Burton's brilliant hard-hitting journalism, coupled with the articulate and vulnerable interviews she did with patients, has created a cultural stir.[14] The important conversation about women's pain and how our system approaches it has been a long time coming. The problem of women's credibility when expressing pain is further exacerbated for women with disabilities.[15]

In the context of the discussion about how best to communicate with doctors, I do not advocate for a tamp down of the emotional aspects of a health journey, which helps nobody and simply play footsie with the *women are hysterical* narrative. Instead, what I believe in is persistence and enlisting the help of someone experienced in advancing the ball in healthcare. When women work together with trusted advocates, more can be accomplished. It isn't that a woman shouldn't cry if that's what she feels like doing; it's getting the right words out through the authentic tears. We can improve the way the system works for ourselves and each other by acknowledging the reality of the injustices that exist and bringing our own truths and powers to the forefront as we communicate with the medical professionals whose job is to support us and help us heal.

TIPS AND TAKEAWAYS

Remember that we are all human actors inside of a complex system with many skewed incentives. Doctors are people with their own set of feelings and stressors.

Take an honest look at the kind of doctor–patient relationship you want as you choose your doctors. Look for the kind of partnership that suits your goals and preferences. Feeling comfortable with your doctors affects your attitude toward your journey.

Engage cordially with your doctors. You don't have to go to great lengths, but letting them know you respect them can enhance your partnership as you take on your health situation.

Spend time preparing for your appointments so that you can be efficient and precise in asking your questions and reporting symptoms and side effects. Practice articulating things with a member of your team so that you become conversant and comfortable.

If you have specific concerns, such as financial worries about affording copayments for procedures or medications, tell your doctor.

Figure out the most seamless and effective way to be in touch with your doctor and medical system when they are busy as well as what to do for emergencies that might arise after hours or on weekends and holidays.

Find out who the right person in your doctor's office or medical system is for different kinds of questions such as scheduling, coverage and treatment protocol. Our system is fragmented and complicated and no one person will have all the answers.

Be mindful and realistic when using the electronic health record and portal system. Answers may not be immediate; you may hear from someone other than your doctor, and you may see imaging reports and test results before your doctor has had the opportunity to review them. If it's helpful to you, have a member of your support/advocacy team check records for you or look with you so that you're not alone in trying to interpret medical jargon or the meaning of something that you may not have the training to interpret.

If you feel that your questions, pain, or concerns are not being addressed to your satisfaction, say so in the moment. While this may be difficult when you are already feeling dismissed, it is important to get past what may be ingrained or unconscious biases that are blocking you from getting the care, treatment, and attention you deserve.

(8)

What to Do If a Bill Is Wrong
or Coverage Is Denied

RECENTLY, I WORKED with a woman in a major northeastern city who was battling a serious illness that required regular blood tests to monitor her condition. She had to change her insurance carrier midstream because the system with which most of her doctors were affiliated dropped her plan. We found her another plan that was accepted by some of the doctors in the system, most importantly the team that was trying to monitor her and refine her diagnosis and treatment options. Over a year later, she called me to tell me that she had gotten a bill for about $800 for blood tests she'd had recently. She assumed she would have to pay the bill. I asked her to send it my way for a look because her routine blood tests had been covered in the past under both her old and new plans.

When I scanned that bill, I knew something was wrong. First, I saw in the top corner that it had been billed under her old plan, which was no longer listed in her portal. I wondered why a system she was treated at so regularly would suddenly revert to billing an old plan. Next, I noticed that the bill did not look like other bills I had seen from the system. The normally colorful logo was black. Where there was usually a reference number that I had come to recognize, this bill had an account number. I called her and told her not to pay the bill just yet because my hackles were up.

In looking carefully at the phone numbers, addresses, and information on the bill, I became concerned that this bill might not be legitimate. I checked her portal and saw that these tests on the dates in question had been listed as billed to her current insurer. On the bill she had been mailed, it said that checks could be sent to an address that had the same PO Box as the medical system's billing center, but in a different zip code. It referred to the name of a lab that I could not find online. It was a generic name tied to the name of the medical system. The phone number listed on the bill said it was "off network" when I called, but then it gave a menu of options anyway, which included calling back during business hours to leave a credit card number or leaving a message for billing questions, which would be answered within forty-eight hours. That seemed strange. The recorded message also referred to a website where patients could go, and when I went there, it would not register the account number listed on the bill when I typed it in, and it led to nonoperating phone numbers and an address that was actually a Pentecostal church in a southern state, not a medical billing office (I checked). I thought this might be a case of fraud, but I could not be sure.

This bill looked plausible, and there is a chance that all that was wrong with it was the insurance that had been billed. But data breaches occur often. As a result, bad actors have patient information, and they know what to do with it. The patient's name and address were correct on the bill, and she had undergone the tests it listed. She had once been covered by the plan listed, though not for some time. I could not ascertain anything for sure, but I was suspicious. Not sure exactly how to proceed, but convinced I should not be Nancy Drewing this matter myself from my phone number and email, I acted on two fronts. I got in touch with a state official, and he had me share paperwork with two lawyers, they ended up passing the matter along to the FBI. I also called legal counsel for the medical system to let him know, figuring that if these bills were being created outside of the system, it could be affecting other patients. The lawyer was helpful and made sure to track the bill from the inside and see if any other patients had reported similar issues.

As for the patient, I told her not to pay the bill. Even if this was not fraud and just extraordinarily confusing, I reasoned, the bill had been submitted to the wrong insurance company and the system would have to resubmit it to the right one. Likely that would mean she would not owe anything. She told me that she was so grateful to the doctors and the medical system that she would absolutely have paid it so as not to anger them, though she is currently unemployed and waiting for disability benefits to be approved. It would have been a hardship, but she was full of gratitude and afraid of being a "problem patient." This impulse is so common. Medical providers know it. Insurance companies know it. Criminals know it.

Bills and Coverage Denials Are Often Incorrect

Even if I resorted to hyperbole, I doubt I could overestimate how often in a woman's health journey something goes wrong that has nothing to do with her prognosis or healing, from unexpected bills to doctors who no longer take her coverage to tests or medications that are strongly recommended yet not preapproved. Recently, a fundraising professional at Bay Area Cancer Connections told me about a client whose doctor recommended a typical protocol for breast cancer treatment. The client's insurer would not preauthorize the treatment, branding it "not reasonable and customary." The doctor called the insurer on the woman's behalf and explained in no uncertain terms that what he was recommending had been the standard of care for over fifteen years. They backed down and approved it immediately. Things like this happen every day. I always counsel women not to assume that a bill or an answer or a denial is correct and to feel safe knowing their coverage cannot be dropped and their premiums cannot be raised because they question and appeal insurance company determinations.

Unfortunately, insurance companies know that many people will not appeal or even investigate their initial decisions, which is why they deny treatments that are not controversial as often as they do. People see an amount owed or a statement of denial in writing and they accept it, granting the insurance companies unearned authority. Women, especially, are conditioned to unquestioningly accept decisions made by officials or executives. There is not much data on how often people pay bills that they should dispute or how often procedures are denied that should be covered, but there is some.

In the realm of Medicare Advantage Plans, for example, claims are routinely denied. According to a 2019 report by the US Department of Health and Human Services Office of Inspector General, fifteen of the top Medicare Advantage plans in the country denied 13 percent of prior authorizations that should have been approved and 18 percent of claims for bills that should have been covered.[1] If this sounds like a cynical money grab that affects potentially vulnerable seniors, that's because it is.

As journalist Marshall Allen posits in his excellent book, *Never Pay the First Bill: And Other Ways to Fight the Health Care System and Win*, our healthcare system is inherently unfair. Allen points out that Americans pay more for healthcare than people in other countries and we do not get our money's worth. He's right. Allen notes that wrong bills are sent often, and our system tolerates fraud. His chapter that shares the book's title, "Never Pay the First Bill," delineates eleven steps that people should go through when they get an incorrect bill.[2] Eleven steps. When a woman is fighting an illness, facing down fear, anxiety, and myriad stressors, she may have to contend with *eleven* steps to follow if she gets a wrong bill. These steps include asking for itemized bills, obtaining records, checking prices, negotiating, crowd-sourcing information, and fine-tooth-combing the Explanation of Benefits that insurers send out after treatments. These are important strategies; smart and well-researched techniques. Allen's book and companion website and videos deliver on their promise to arm people with tools to protect themselves from a predatory system, and I'm grateful he has done this work. One of his eleven steps is to find a patient advocate. For women, as this entire book attests, I think this should be step one.

Stay Organized for an Appeal

Because questionable denials are common, every woman should be prepared to start an appeal process, preferably with help. Staying organized is key. The top-line details to focus on are the reason for the denial, the parties who will review the appeal, the deadlines for filing, and the timeline for an insurance company response. Lining up doctors to communicate that what they are recommending is the *standard of care* will be crucial if an appeal is necessary. If this holds up a woman's treatment, which it can, she can ask the doctor whether there is a clinical trial in progress that she can join to avoid more delays.

In some cases, insurance companies will expedite appeals. These situations include when your doctor believes waiting would affect maximum possible recovery or subject a woman to severe pain. In cases of cancer and other serious illnesses, this is often arguable, and I tell women to specifically state that their appeal is urgent. I've also seen women in the middle of hospital stays resort to urgent appeals. The turnaround time is twenty-four to seventy-two hours, and I advise women not to hesitate to ask unless a treatment has already been received and denied. As a last resort, if appeals have been exhausted, a woman can also ask for something called an *external review*. This is where a third party, outside of the insurance company, looks at the facts and decides whether or not the insurance company's denial was appropriate. If the third party finds the insurance should cover the claim, the insurance company must do so. An appeal is basically a conversation between parties to a contract, patient and insurer, who do not agree. An external review is akin to taking that disagreement to arbitration. Very few of the women I help have ever heard of an external review, but according to the Patient Empowerment Network, patients are successful about half the time they ask for one.[3] Those are good odds.

When things like coverage decisions go wrong for women, the socio-emotional piece to the puzzle needs to be addressed. It's a gating item because this system is full of bills, chills, and last-minute stressors and causes women considerable anxiety.

I am reminded of a story about a lovely, smart, and thorough woman named Annie who was going in for some pre-op for breast cancer surgery on a Tuesday after a holiday weekend. Annie had solid insurance and a hopeful outlook because of early detection, but she could not get the preauthorization answers she needed, and it was Friday afternoon when we first spoke. People seemed to be gone from their desks, and she could not get a call back, though she had been trying all week. The stress on her, worrying about getting billed for an unanticipated out-of-network specialist or something else unforeseen, agitated her. Frankly, it ruined a weekend that should have been spent relaxing and preparing for what she was about to undergo.

Annie made every call, sent every email, and messaged inside her portals, but nobody answered her. Not the medical system, the insurers, the human resources department of the employer who provided the coverage—nobody. So she went into her pre-op procedure, frazzled instead of comfortable and prepared. I tried to reassure her that I found it hard to believe that medical personnel would put the oxygen mask over her face in the operating room on Tuesday morning if the procedure had not been greenlit in time. I believed that somebody would let her know. I hope those assurances alleviated some of her anxiety, but I cannot blame her for being worried. It should not go like this, but so often it does. So many women fear getting bills that will sink them or set them back. Whether a big bill comes early on or well after treatment, it's always an ill-timed and unnerving distraction.

The No Surprises Act Unpacked

There has been some good legislative news on this front in the form of a recent federal law known as the No Surprises Act, though it was the product of politicized negotiations and is not completely watertight. On its face, the idea behind the law, which became effective at the start of 2022, is that consumers should be protected from surprise medical bills when they receive care, whether or not the care is in an emergency setting. The idea is that if a patient does not have control over the care they receive, they should not have a bill sprung upon them and should be charged as though the care received was in-network under whatever plan they have. But nothing is that simple. For example, in the realm of emergencies, helicopters are covered, but ground ambulances are not because those services are controlled by local governments.[4] This makes no intuitive sense, of course, and it invites gouging by ground ambulance companies unless state regulators remain focused and vigilant. Furthermore, Medicare patients should be covered for emergency helicopter transports, but if they have opted out of paying for that coverage, they can still be charged. When you consider the nature of an emergency, you can imagine that a person in need of this service might not efficiently communicate or be asked about a Medicare opt-out. Loophole alert.

COVID-19 made telehealth common, though the technology was available before 2020 (much like Zoom). One story sticks out as a cautionary tale that illustrates more of the limits of the No Surprises Act. A New York woman returned home from an overseas trip in September 2022 with congestion and sinus pain. To be considerate of others, she thought she should try a telehealth appointment with her regular medical system. All of her doctors accepted her insurance. The doctor she spoke with quickly ruled out Covid, decided she had a sinus infection, and prescribed an antibiotic and steroid nasal spray. According to the patient, the entire interaction took about five minutes, yet she was billed $660 for a "45–59 minute visit."[5] Her insurance denied the whole amount, claiming the visit to have been out-of-network. It turned out that the specific doctor who picked up the call did not accept her coverage, though she had been told that the estimated out-of-pocket would be about sixty dollars.

Here's the kicker: though the No Surprises Act is supposed to protect someone who gets charged for out-of-network charges that they did not know were out-out-of-network (hence the name of the act), these rules apply when an out-of-network provider charges a patient for care received *at* a facility that is in-network. Telehealth is not *at* any facility, so the insurer claimed it was unclear whether it was a facility in-network, even though it was part of a medical system that was.[6] If this gives you a headache (which the patient in question already had), I advise that you make a call to the medical provider before you log into a telehealth appointment to make sure that it will be covered by your insurance. Additionally, there's the whole question of signing consent to be charged uncovered overages, which patients routinely do in order to be treated, but suffice it to say that even with laws written with patient protection at the purported forefront, there are exceptions and workarounds that insurers know how to exploit.

"Shopping" for Healthcare

For about a decade as of this writing, there has been a push toward "price transparency" and ensuing comparison shopping. Patients have begun to understand that they are also consumers, and watchdog organizations have cropped up to assist. Sites such as www.healthcarebluebook.com allow users to plug in procedures or treatments and their zip code to see "fair prices" for them. Granted, there's the free site and then the premium site, which gives more detailed information for a fee (some employers provide it as a benefit for their employees), another example of companies profiting from the mess we're in. With medical costs and fear spiraling out of control, price transparency is still a good development. It helps in the decision-making phases, and it can also be helpful when something goes wrong. For example, if a medical system is willing to negotiate a bill after coverage has been denied, it is extremely useful to be able to access actual average costs in a region. Women can be empowered by information as they go through treatment for serious illness. In the age of data and information, it helps to know how to access the valuable tools that exist.

TIPS AND TAKEAWAYS

Female patients already feel vulnerable interacting with a medical system that is not designed for them. When something goes wrong, it is especially stressful, and they often assume they must pay incorrect bills or make impossible choices. I have my own checklist for women when something goes wrong outside of medical issues themselves. I've gone over these steps with women I advocate for well over a thousand times. Prior to writing this book, I have never had occasion to write it down.

1. Find someone to act as your advocate. (If you don't have anyone, I volunteer.)

2. Make sure you have itemized paperwork documenting the denial of the claim or authorization. (If not, ask for it, both from the provider and the insurance company.)

3. Check for things on the paperwork that look irregular. (Was it billed to the right plan? Are the codes consistent with the diagnosis? If it's a bill, were all the billed services provided?)

4. Call the insurance company and ask them to verify the statement.

5. Tell your provider that your insurance company has issued a denial. (They will often negotiate a lower price if they see that it is not covered.)

6. If you are employed or covered by an employer-provided plan, ask the human resources department to advocate on your behalf or guide you.

7. Check into disease-specific patient support programs or emergency funds.

8. Investigate the appeals process. (It's usually on the website of the insurance company. Calling them to be directed to it will work too.)

9. If you are having trouble getting access to care, ask if there is a case advocate inside the insurance company available or a hospital social worker who can assist you.

10. Check with nurses or administrative employees in your doctor's office about whether they can help you make sense of what went wrong.

11. Talk directly with the billing department at the provider who sent the bill or denial.

It turns out I have eleven steps, too, which is not what I expected. I thought it would be fewer, but each of these is more like a door to a potential waterfall of questions that can arise. When things go wrong it can fill a woman with righteous indignation. It feels unjust, and it is healthy for women to stand up for themselves. Maybe your case won't be the case that finally makes the world stand up and notice how broken the system is, but at least you can protect yourself during your healing journey and come back in fighting shape.

COMMON REASONS FOR HEALTH INSURANCE DENIALS

These are reasons that routinely appear on form denial letters. In every case, I tell women their first call should be to the doctor or medical system that submitted the claim to ask for support. They have seen it all before and usually have information at their fingertips to help with next steps.

- Care not medically necessary
- Care not appropriate in healthcare setting or level of care
- Effectiveness of treatment not proven
- Treatment considered experimental
- Claim improperly filed

WHAT TO DO IF PRESCRIBED MEDICATION IS NOT COVERED

- Ask your doctor if there is an alternative that might be covered.
- Seek out generics.
- Request an exception from your insurer.
- Look into copayment, coupons, and assistance plans from the company that makes the drug.

❨ 9 ❩

Creative Solutions and Mindfulness

YEARS AGO, I worked with a woman named Monica. She learned of her breast cancer diagnosis four months after she had been laid off from her job, and she had declined COBRA coverage because it was prohibitively expensive. Monica was concerned that the only individual health insurance she could buy was not going to cover the doctors she hoped to be treated by. So, after a wide-ranging conversation, she decided to turn her knitting hobby and side hustle into an organized online business with a few friends. They sold products, gave online classes, and created a space for other people to show and sell their knitwear. Because they were now employed by the small company, they were able to purchase group health insurance. Monica got the best coverage available to support her ongoing health journey. All because of creative problem-solving.

Prioritize Mental Health and Be Open to Creative Problem-Solving

When you're facing an illness, you will be focused on the facts and statistics applicable to your physical health. It's always a puzzle. Part of the process is prioritizing your mental well-ness too. It's imperative that you don't expend much needed energy on fear and anxiety. One of the ways I have worked with women who need support is to brainstorm creative solutions when work, money, insurance, or other worries preoc-cupy them. The practice of collaborative problem-solving can make you feel seen, heard, and cared for. And thinking cre-atively is empowering.

Thinking about how you can be covered may not seem like the most creative endeavor. It's not exactly the stuff of vision boarding or decoupage, but I have seen it make a dif-ference. In chapter 4, I discussed the reasons that staying on a group health insurance plan may be the most affordable and secure way to go through a health journey. Before the Affordable Care Act, it was difficult for women with serious illnesses to get individual health insurance coverage at all. The key in those days, as I always advised women, was to be on a group plan at all costs. Today, individual coverage is available through state exchanges for anyone who can pay for it, regard-less of their health status. However, group health insurance plans are still more affordable and tend to have better coverage because the risks are spread. Both before and after the pas-sage of the Affordable Care Act, I've worked with women who either could not attain individual coverage or were unable to afford it. More than once, an out-of-the-box creative solution was the answer. Monica's story is just one among many others. For example, professionals like realtors, hairdressers, actors, and writers tend to be self-employed. Some have high enough incomes to pay for individual policies, but many do not. Often, they will do well to consider joining a trade or business organization in their field that provides a group health insurance option. This is something I have always been surprised to find people don't usually think about. In other circumstances, a person may be a freelancer who can band together with others who work in the same field, form a business, and become eligible to purchase a group health insurance plan.

Another example of creativity is an open mind about what one would be willing to pay for out-of-pocket in the information-gathering phase of treatment. I often advise people to pay cash if they can for consultations or second opinions. Even if a person is insured or a member of a Health Maintenance Organization like Kaiser Permanente, second opinions are something to spend on if they are not covered or are only partially covered, because they are finite and high value. No procedures and no prescriptions. If a woman is uninsured and being treated at a state or county facility for free, paying for a second opinion could also be worthwhile. It allows a woman to access experience and knowledge about treatment options and possible protocols for the price of one appointment. Once she knows what her protocol should be, it could be more than adequate to receive the treatments and medications from the provider where she is best covered. Sticking with the most comprehensive plan may not apply as easily to surgeries. But where there are other questions to be asked and answered, such as how many procedures the doctor has done or rates of success, it works well for non-surgical treatment decisions. The guiding principle is to be flexible about paying for expert advice. If paying for an appointment is not feasible, grants, subsidies, or sliding scale fees could be available. It is always worth it to ask, and often prices will be different once a provider learns that there is no third-party payer involved and payment will be direct from the patient.

Creative Thinking in the Workplace and Beyond

Creative thinking can also happen in the workplace, and these stories seldom get told. Once I worked with a woman named Rita who did not want to go on disability full-time, though her doctor felt that she would qualify because of her medical situation. She wanted to stay active and engaged and enjoyed her job and colleagues, but she knew that full-time work was going to be out of the question for a while. Rita was worried about asking her employer to accommodate her with a flexible part-time schedule, even if that was likely her legal right, because she knew it was complicated to work out and that they needed full-time people to serve their client base. We brainstormed and came up with an unconventional idea. Rita approached human resources at her large company and asked if there were any other employees doing similar work who might be open to job-share, either due to health needs or childcare responsibilities. It seemed like a pie-in-the-sky request, but we felt she had little to lose because she knew she'd qualify for disability. It turned out there was a woman in Rita's department out on maternity leave who only wanted to come back part-time and had asked about it, but with low hopes that it would work out. Amazingly, the company was willing to "match" these women up, keep them both on the company health insurance plan, and retain two trained and loyal employees. This had nothing to do with applicable laws; it was simply an out-of-the-ordinary question to ask. In the post-Covid world, possibilities like this may be more available because though there is a trend toward returning to in-person work, the work-from-home genie is out of the bottle and has normalized workplace flexibility and creative solutions.

Another instance of creative thinking was less successful but is nonetheless instructive. It involved real estate. I got a call from Bay Area Cancer Connections one day in the late 2010s, asking if I could chat with a woman named Ella who was late-stage in her cancer journey and out of income sources. She was concerned that she'd have to sell her home. Ella was sixty years old and not working, as her illness didn't allow for that any longer. She was able to access Medicaid coverage because she was disabled, but her SSI disability payments were not enough to help her with copayments, food, and other expenses. Her condominium was worth about $1.5 million. According to her prognosis, Ella expected to live for a year or two and had a peaceful and positive outlook. We went through the list of other options for income supplementation—things like grants from national cancer organizations, hardship distributions from pension plans, and life insurance policies that could be accessed for cash value, but nothing clicked.

Ella and I put our heads together. We talked through her priorities and goals. Ella did not have children and was not concerned about leaving her home to anyone, but she wanted to live out her days there. She was open to any arrangement that could help her do that. With that, we each reached out to some realtor friends to see if they had any buyers or investors who would want to lock in an under-market price and let her stay so she could access the cash she needed to live on. They all said the same thing: even if it's a bargain, nobody wants to buy a house under those circumstances. It broke my heart that people could think that way. I can remember my real estate lawyer father telling me stories about people in New York City reading the obituaries to scope out available apartments in tight markets. Maybe that was cold and opportunistic, but it acknowledged the reality of the life/death continuum.

I dug further and came up with what I thought was a creative and reasonable idea—what if we could talk a bank into giving Ella a reverse mortgage? She was more than amenable, and I knew retirees did this all the time. A reverse mortgage is a loan extended to a homeowner in exchange for an equity share in the property. The loan does not have to be repaid in real time; it is usually payable when the homeowner sells, moves, or passes away. We both wondered if the concept could be extended to someone who was ill. Ella's life expectancy was possibly more predictable than someone simply over a certain age. With her cooperation, I called every person I knew in real estate, mortgage lending, and home appraisals. None of them had ever heard of a reverse mortgage in the case of someone terminally ill. We found out this is because the banks will not do it. The Federal Housing Authority set the eligible age for reverse mortgages at sixty-two, and banks won't make exceptions because they need to be able to turn around and sell their loans to be packaged back up into mortgage-backed securities. Nobody will buy a loan that doesn't fit inside the Federal Housing Authority guardrails; it will just sit there on the bank's balance sheet. It simply isn't worth the trouble for a bank to make a loan like this one.

After over twenty-five years of helping women with cancer get through their treatments, hold on to their jobs, access benefits, and tap resources for money when they need it, I have learned a lot about what works and what might be more of a goose chase, but I don't always guess right. In the case of this real estate plan gone awry, it is true that it took time and effort. The idea didn't work. But I spent time with Ella, and we became friends and creative problem solvers on a mutual mission. We learned. This could be an avenue for cancer organizations to lobby for legislation at the state and federal level, and I've spoken to many real estate professionals who agree. It could also be a place for compassionate investment that's good for all the parties. Not a waste of time, not mine nor Ella's.

When someone receives a diagnosis, typically their first thought is to find the best doctors. Doctors who have treated the most patients, surgeons with the most experience. In a well-functioning system, this would always make sense. But there is so much more complexity, and while I understand the temptation to go all ostrich about it, because it is deeply convoluted and can be depressing, I'm advocating for a better way. The way of enlightened skepticism and widening the lens to think expansively. I approach patient and workplace advocacy both methodically and creatively. I listen to the client first and hear about what is on her mind and what help she thinks she needs. I consider work, health, family situations, available benefits, geography, and finances.

After the reverse mortgage idea was shot down, we were able to find local cancer-relief grants through Bay Area Cancer Connections to support Ella's journey. Ella and I discussed the reverse mortgage concept with the executive director and some key staff members, and now tapping the value of real estate is on the front burner for us as a new way to help our clients navigate their paths. And reverse mortgages for people who are terminally ill is an avenue to pursue legislatively that might make an important difference for some people.

Creative thinking can take women far when they are fighting illness, and it can also give them purpose, social connection, and a feeling that what they do matters, as they could perhaps pave the way for someone in a similar situation. Looking ahead and defining goals is the first step. Considering possibly overlooked factors that can affect eligibility for benefits, legal protection, health insurance, and financial help can take you far and keep you calm.

The "M" Word: Mindfulness

Then, there's the internal creative work, the work of mindfulness. Mindfulness has become a mainstay of fridge magnets and greeting cards, and that should be a clue that deeper consideration is warranted. The concept is so often bandied about and commoditized in our culture that it can be hard to know what it means, much less how to effectively practice it.

When it comes to the mindfulness movement, which is unregulated, there is a lot to unpack, but it's worth the effort. To get meta about it, women facing illness should be mindful about mindfulness. There is so much information out there— so many apps, memes, social media accounts, podcasters, and bloggers—that, ironically, a notion centered on how to gain clarity and simplicity can get overwhelming. I have found that permission to question and fashion one's own path creatively are key.

The first thing to be thoughtful about is the danger of toxic positivity. Bookshelves and media are full of uplifting, inspiring, and articulate messaging about ways to create the life we want, and *staying positive* is always a watchword. As statements and research get watered down and turned into sound bites and self-proclaimed gurus abound and profit, it can become difficult and even lonely for women who find themselves facing illness because of the certain and monolithic tone of what they sometimes read, see, and hear. Positivity sells. But when people who are not facing illness insist upon the always sunny as the only way forward for a healthy, productive life, it can make women facing illness feel excluded and misunderstood. The "good vibes only" train has left the station, and it can make people who are challenged by illness feel left behind and othered.[1] The fix is to find sensitive, specific mindfulness practices that are thorough, not reductive. The good news is that they exist.

The oversimplification of the notion of manifestation, which is a widespread but not always deeply understood idea, presents another challenge. New age teachers and thinkers tout that people attract the energy they give off, that thinking something can make it so, and that people make themselves sick by indulging in negativity and not releasing their anger and fear appropriately. You can see how it this might go sideways for a woman diagnosed with a serious illness. I've had women call me crying because they feel overwhelmed by the sense that somehow what they're going through is their fault. That they attracted or created their illness.

Additionally, many of these messages have been co-opted by materialism, as though the skill of a mindfulness athlete is measured by a sports car conjured into a garage or some other financial windfall. These ideas may effectively fuel ambitions and life paths for some, but they can have regrettable unintended consequences that can hurt women when they're dealing with the strains and stresses of an illness. Mindfulness reduced can feel like another societal pressure that makes women feel inadequate.

But effective mindfulness goes beyond oversimplified positivity or formulaic manifestation. It is staying present, a Buddhist style of observation and living in the moment. It's being where you are and noticing the beauty and brilliance around you. It is not categorically or proscriptively Pollyannaish, though the practice has been shown to evoke positive feelings. These effects are borne out by medical research.[2] Mindfulness is helpful for people facing chronic illness because mindfulness:

- Encourages self-care
- Helps people stop defining themselves based on their illness
- Helps people embrace their own humanness
- Increases receptivity to expanded healing options
- May help people let go of the original life they planned
- Aids gratitude
- Helps silence the inner critic, and pave the way for compassion[3]

When a woman is facing a serious illness, these are no small things. Authentic joy is powerful, and women facing illness do well to get past the noise and explore mindfulness on their own terms.

There are many modalities and practices that work to help people get through difficulty, find peace and solace, and even, in some cases, heal. The trick for women who are facing illness is to find the right outlets, practitioners, mindfulness techniques, and community to serve their needs. At Bay Area Cancer Connections, as well as many sister organizations around the country, tailored mindfulness programming is available. In my experience, organizations that support women on their health journeys are the optimal place to start, as there are so many options (e.g., community centers, spas, gyms, apps) that aren't vetted in terms of the expertise of the leaders or are just too broad or untargeted. It also helps to be among people who are having similar experiences, as it builds community and understanding. It is much less likely that someone will say or do something that will have a negative effect on your emotions and mindset.

Some of the many mindfulness options available are meditation, guided imagery, journaling, aromatherapy, music immersion, yoga, Tai Chi, progressive muscle relaxation, and nature experiences. This is just a short list, and finding the right mindfulness mix for yourself can be a healthy exercise of self-discovery all its own. Experimentation, learning and openness to growth are potent creative portals.

Mindfulness is only a part of effective mental health. Many enlightening books have been written about psychiatry and psychology. Most medical systems, women's health centers, and disease-specific organizations have lists of excellent therapists who specialize in treating women who are working through illness. It is always worthwhile to explore your options and find the best mental healthcare for your situation and needs. A person dedicated to helping you process your unvarnished fears and concerns can be instrumental, as it may be hard to share these feelings with people you love or those dependent on you. It may be that your partner, closest family members, and friends can benefit from this kind of help as well, so that you can all pull together and function as the strongest team possible.

TIPS AND TAKEAWAYS

There is more than one way to stay covered, find financial support, and thrive while fighting illness. A key to combating hopelessness is to look at things from more than one perspective. The following examples are ideas that aren't typical first lines of thinking but have proven useful to women when they are battling illness.

If health insurance is a concern for you and you don't have a group plan through your employer or your spouse's employer, consider where there any other ways you might become part of a group through professional affiliations, trade or business associations, or by joining up with others.

If you're taking time out from work and taking classes in-person or online, that could be another unexplored route to joining a group. Check on the prices and coverage of available individual plans and compare.

If you own your home and are over sixty-two years old, you can consider a reverse mortgage to alleviate financial pressures.

If you own a home with more than one bedroom, you can supplement your income by renting your space, possibly through a home-sharing platform.

If you live near a teaching hospital, investigate whether a medical or nursing school has a rental listing service for their students. You could end up with a wonderful tenant and supplement your income.

If you work for a company with dedicated human resources, schedule a meeting and explore whether they have any flexibility outside of the legal requirements and formal employee benefits programs for employees as they fight illness.

If you have a life insurance policy, it may have a disability benefit that you haven't pursued, and if you need cash, that could be a source you haven't considered. Not all life insurance policies have disability benefits, but some have redeemable cash value.

If you've saved retirement funds in a 401(k) or other tax-preferred vehicle, investigate whether or not there are disability or hardship provisions that allow you access to your money without penalty.

Mindfulness options abound at every price point, including free. Here are some things to consider as you fashion the right formula for yourself:

Meditation takes many forms and there are many free meditations available on apps, YouTube, and the Web. Traditional transcendental meditation is widely taught and is a practice that can be done anywhere once you have found your mantra and learned how to meditate with a certified instructor. Guided imagery is a simple meditation technique that has been shown to relax both body and mind. It is effective for pain reduction.[4]

Even before the pandemic, online classes and communities centered around practicing mindfulness were worldwide. Check in with your local women's wellness center or disease-specific organization first to see what they have available. It is also possible to connect with other women through organizations like AARP, the American Cancer Society, the American Heart Association, and smaller organizations that create mindfulness spaces and programs for their members.

Journaling has proven mental health benefits, including reducing anxiety and depression and increasing awareness and emotional regulation. It has even been shown to speed up physical healing in certain circumstances.[5]

There are myriad programs, prompts, and pre-printed options for journaling. I've been a storytelling coach for over twenty years. Over this time, I've developed some writing prompts specifically for women who are on health journeys. The following have been particularly useful:

1. Describe the woman that you are. Then, describe the woman you want to be. If there are gaps, talk about ways you can bridge them.

2. Put together a list of ten to fifteen songs that constitute the soundtrack of your life. Under each one, explain how it makes you feel and the lyric you often repeat or sing in your head.

3. What moments from your childhood most formed the woman that you are today?

4. If your heart has not healed from the way someone hurt you, write that person a letter and tell them why.

5. If you want forgiveness from someone, write a letter explaining how you feel.

6. Write about your responsibilities and how they make you feel.

7. Write with specificity about what brings you joy and why.

8. Visualize healing and write about what it looks like to you.

9. Write about a perfect, peaceful day.

10. Write a mission statement for your life. What is your purpose, and what steps you will take to achieve it?

11. When it comes to your life experience, what makes you proud?

12. Write about some moments from books, movies, or other media that are touchstones for you. Why do you think you keep going back to them in your mind?

13. Describe what you react to when you look at art and how it makes you feel.

❮ 10 ❯

What Is the Real Problem?

WHEN I FOUND myself facing secondary infertility of unex-
plained etiology, my husband worked for a firm that had amazing health insurance. It covered in vitro fertilization (IVF),
which was highly unusual. We would not have been able to
afford it otherwise. My mother was beside herself with worry
as I considered this route because she'd just been through a
breast cancer battle. She was terrified of me taking large doses
of powerful hormones, fearful that they might shake loose
some predisposition toward cancer that was embedded in my
cells. I understood and shared those anxieties, but I managed
them as best I could. I didn't know at the time that my sister
would later be diagnosed with breast cancer as well and that
I'd worry more about the risk I took as a result. I also already
had a beautiful, intelligent, and kind daughter (my firstborn),
and there was a good argument that I should have let the chips
fall where they might, that I would either conceive after an
even larger gap of time or be grateful for the lovely "one and
done" family that I had. But I was gripped. The beat of the
mother drum reverberated, and it was all I could hear. I had
the chance, so I took it.

Being an IVF patient changed me. I learned deep lessons about love, loss, faith, control, compassion, pain, guilt, loneliness, and grace. I experienced what it feels like to be a patient, to temper hope with realism. I made new friends, connected by a common struggle that bound us together. I became sensitized to the offhand comments people made about how easily they got pregnant, and the questions people casually asked one another about their plans as though such a blessing were a given. I became a more positively sensitized mother too. Every second felt beautifully rare, and the tedious parts receded. Today, I know what a gift my adult daughters are, though the journey of bringing each of them into existence could not have been more different.

After two cycles of stimulation and egg retrieval and a successful transfer, we had fertilized embryos left over. They were frozen and stored in a cryochamber at the hospital where I'd had the IVF, where my daughter was born, where she stopped breathing and her heart stopped pumping in the neonatal intensive care unit at the age of three weeks, and where she was revived. If those walls could talk. Sometimes, during long sleepless nights during her illness, I felt they did. The decision to freeze those embryos was made just after implantation, and I can't say I thought this part of the process through. I felt grateful that I had successful retrievals, that I was young and had gotten pregnant, and I had no idea what was to come. It never occurred to me that I'd have frozen embryos to consider across town. But I did. My husband didn't want more children. After nearly losing our second baby girl when she was a newborn, he felt his heart could take no more. I understood, though there was a part of me that wanted to keep having babies, and as some kind of emotional crutch I kept those embryos frozen for years. It cost money, and every time the renewal bill came around, I felt conflicted. Finally, when my younger daughter was a teen and I was involved with breast cancer screenings and then an ovarian surgery, it was time to decide what to do. It was hard, and the options were few. We decided that if we donated the embryos to scientific research, perhaps our struggles would yield better health or a medical advance that might help others. It never occurred to me that this was controversial, though considering recent developments I know differently now. It was a personal decision, and certainly not one that I took lightly.

The paperwork for donating the embryos was over-the-top, even for me. I confess that while I understood the complexities that the lawyers were drafting against, things like donors having no right to know about the research or its results, I could not bear to read what I was signing. Once I made what I thought was the right decision, I wanted to be finished. I had miscarried twice, the second time my daughter's twin. It had been a bittersweet journey. As I recall, the bill to keep the embryos frozen and stored was something like $600 a year. After the donation was processed and the frozen embryos were brought to the lab, I went through my own kind of mourning, private and quiet. I tried not to let it consume me. Fortunately, my hands and heart were full of love and life.

Then the past-due bills notices began to arrive. Repeatedly, I called the hospital system billing department. After hours on hold, I explained anew that the embryos were no longer being stored and that they had been donated to a lab at the adjacent medical school. The answer was always the same, that it would be rectified. But for a year, the bills came like clockwork, hurting my heart, though I knew full well that it had nothing to do with me. Even with the late charges, I could have saved a lot of valuable time by simply paying, and that's clearly what the hospital system was optimizing for. But I kept disputing the bill, making calls, sending emails, and writing letters because it was a matter of principle. I was a patient advocate and had to stand for making sure billing systems were held accountable.

What happened next shocked me. The hospital billing system, the same one that had assured me month after month, sent the bill to collections, and now an agency was after us daily and our credit rating was at risk. For a bill that should have been zeroed out. For a service not rendered. After we'd made a wrenching but philanthropic choice for the good of humanity. How predatory and absurd. It took a barn burner of a lawyer letter to the hospital system, threatening swift legal action, to call off the dogs for good. A fiery, combative piece, and I took no joy in that exchange, but it was necessary.

Healthcare Is a Business

This is how our system functions. The squeezing of dollars, the wearing down of patients, the layers of bureaucracy, and the managing of care. It's a shell game, as third-party reimbursements are determined by algorithms, actuarial tables and betting tactics that you would expect to be reserved for hedge funds. Because hospitals and doctors are reimbursed according to Wild West rules, they continue to charge more or stop doing business with certain insurers altogether. The dynamic is destabilizing and destructive. The system never reaches equilibrium, and it is ultimately the patients who pay, fiscally and psychically.

In a nutshell, the problem that we all face with our current medical system—that women bear the disproportionate brunt of—is institutionalized, systemic greed. Extreme bottom-lining. What shocks me most is how normalized this has become. Good people scratch our heads, shrug our shoulders, and heave a collective "that's capitalism in America" sigh. The medical-industrial complex is an affiliation of profit-making and purportedly nonprofit entities, but the system's incentives, innovations, devices, drugs, and adjacent services run on dollars. With management consultants and private equity involved, as they are in many instances, the layers of greed, which I define here as relentless profit maximization, have created a hamster wheel of hardship for many patients. In a field where healing humans is the goal, this is simply incongruous, yet it has ossified.

As Dr. Elizabeth Rosenthal wrote in her groundbreaking 2017 book, *An American Sickness: How Healthcare Became a Big Business and How You Can Take It Back*, there is no single culprit here. There are many.[1] Hospitals, drug companies, medical device makers, some doctors, and medically adjacent companies (like ambulance services providers) are not resistant to greed. The morals of the marketplace, such as they are, govern. Treatments, guidelines, medications, and testing are all subject to the laws of commerce.

Dr. Lisa Cook, an internal medicine expert who has worked with infectious diseases, including hepatitis, explains that most hospital systems have purchased a specialized ultrasound machine called a FibroScan, which allows doctors to test the extent of liver scarring in patients. It's a fast test which yields immediate results and it's a cheaper and less invasive procedure than liver biopsies. Most FibroScans are charged out at under $500, whereas liver biopsies cost over $6000. But it turns out that the results of FibroScans are subjective and variable and that simple more affordable blood tests that cost around $60 are just as reliable. Dr. Cook said that the lack of reliability in FibroScans is especially pronounced for patients who are obese or have ascites or metabolic syndrome, which are common in people who have liver scarring. But once the purchase has been made, the machine must be used, and the insurance will be billed. Doctors order the tests, and insurers reimburse because it's cheaper than doing biopsies. But it still costs the system. Does this help patients in terms of their health outcomes when they are having the pertinent blood tests anyway? Not necessarily. This is just one example of how standards set for reasons other than patient outcomes become common protocol.

Dr. Donald Berwick is the former president and CEO of the Institute for Healthcare Improvement. He has written and spoken extensively about the corrosive effect of greed on our system. Dr. Berwick brilliantly breaks down the chain of greed, pointing to the pharmaceutical companies' monopolistic corner on the drug market, health insurers who consistently buck reimbursements and obfuscate and complicate billing procedures, predatory hospital pricing, health inequities borne of providers favoring wealthy populations over low-income groups, outsized salaries and benefits for executives in the healthcare industry, and corporate transactions such as mergers and acquisitions that benefit profiteers. As Dr. Berwick puts it, "kleptocapitalist behaviors that raise prices, salaries, market power, and government payment to extreme levels hurt patients and families, vulnerable institutions, governmental programs, small and large businesses, and workforce morale."[2]

At a high level, the stock market tells a story. In the next chapter, I will explain in detail how our system got to where it is from a historical perspective. But for now, a peek into the S&P 500 reveals a stark truth: healthcare stocks as a category rank second in terms of revenue and profits, behind only the technology sector.[3] The healthcare category includes pharmaceutical companies, medical equipment and device companies, and entities that conduct medical research. These stocks are considered noncyclical, meaning regardless of the economic climate, up or down, consumers will spend money in this sector.[4] For-profit hospitals, dialysis centers, imaging centers, rehab facilities, and in-home health companies are largely investor-backed.[5] Healthcare is a huge business, an engine of prosperity for investors. And the hypergrowth ethos reaches beyond the for-profit sector. Most nonprofits in the healthcare space must engage in marketing and advertising to stay afloat.[6] The pressures are real and bad actors abound.[7] The poorest and most vulnerable patients are hounded with bills[8], and fraud and exploitation are increasingly common.[9] On the executive compensation side, CEO pay in the healthcare space rounds out the picture. The CEOs of CVS Health, Aetna, United Health Group, and Cigna each earn over $20 million per year.[10] Executives work hard and take risks, sure. But when doctors are wondering if their patients will be covered for treatments and diagnostic tests they feel are needed, and when they are being choked by premiums, this should raise eyebrows and concerns.[11] But it is what happens when greed rules.

The Role of Big Pharma

The Big Pharma piece of the puzzle has been well documented. Beth Macy's hard-hitting book, *Dopesick: Dealers, Doctors, and the Drug Company That Addicted America,* exposed the abject greed of Purdue Pharma and its owners, doctors, and employees who got caught up in the madness. As the book expressed and the Hulu series dramatized, this not only made people rich off the suffering of others, it cost many lives.[12] Recently, drugmakers Eli Lilly and Novo Nordisk have been raking in billions on weight loss drugs.[13] Mounjaro and Zepbound, Ozempic and Wegovy are sought-after and not often covered by insurance. At a moment of potential medical breakthroughs in the fight against obesity, many women who could benefit from these drugs will not be able to access them because they are not covered by Medicaid, Medicare, or less expensive insurance plans. If they were, it would ultimately save our healthcare system billions in treatments for conditions that are an outgrowth of obesity. Rich people will buy the drugs for cash, as we have already seen play out in Hollywood. Big Pharma and its investors will be enriched. Even if more competition and better coverage eventually ensues, which is likely, it is a short-run gold rush that will be capitalized upon.

Health-Related Products and Services

In an earlier chapter, I talked about the effect of electronic health records on patient care and patient-doctor communication, but there's more to say when it comes to greed. These systems are just one example of administrative costs that ultimately get passed on to patients. There are layers of products and services adjacent to healthcare that are positioned to provide a revenue stream for founders and backers. Medical devices and technology solutions abound. From specialized syringes to ultrasound gel warmers, the innovations continue. While there's no question that scientists and businesspeople are working hard to improve patient outcomes and that many have the best of intentions, it is also true that most of the entities they work for are investor-backed, and the pressure to create lucrative outcomes is pronounced.

Insurance Companies

Insurance companies do their own profit maximization, and it can be egregious. This subject has already been touched on in this book because it is a dominant problem. It presents in specific ways. To start, the process of prior authorization. It is used as a significant bureaucratic challenge to the delivery of important care when it is needed. Another thing health insurers do is a "fail first" technique when it comes to approving expensive medications. Doctors and patients are often forced to use cheaper drugs first and prove that they didn't work before more effective but more expensive solutions are approved. Perhaps the biggest avenue that medical insurance companies use in denying treatment is the "medical necessity" standard. Because it can be elastic and the facts of each case are often different, insurance companies invoke this in an overinclusive way and it costs patients precious time and stresses the system. The US Department of Health and Human Services did a study in 2022, which shockingly found that 13 percent of Medicare Advantage denials by commercial insurers should have been covered.[14] This kind of systemic gaming is what caused journalist Marshall Allen to research and write his book *Never Pay the First Bill: And Other Ways to Fight the Health Care System and Win*, which I discussed earlier.[15] The cumbersome appeals process costs our system money, no question.[16] I cannot accurately count the times I have assured a woman I'm advocating for that a bill or a denial she has gotten along the way on her journey to wellness is not the final word. We're stuck with market-based realities, and yet we saddle ourselves with such inefficiency.

Advocacy for Women Works

Because of my work, I look at this through the lens of women's wellness. The stories of "pay out-of-pocket or go without" have hit so many of the women I have advocated for. The time and energy I have spent attempting to make things right that should never have gone wrong is hard to fathom. When we take a holistic look at our system of healthcare and who it hurts most, I know it was worth it in every single case. I see that this greed and the medical apartheid that it engenders makes women feel unimportant, locked out, and irrelevant.

What I have come to understand is that every woman needs a guide, an advocate, a sounding board, and a second pair of eyes and ears. People have asked me repeatedly why this book is for women, and I've got chapter and verse answers about why women are more categorically disadvantaged by the system, but there's something else I have realized in working with so many women as they face illness. Often women are givers, nurturers, and community builders. This system was not built for people who approach the world from those vantage points. It is made of meaner stuff. In fact, the eat-or-be-eaten ethos of American healthcare is so extreme that to many women, interacting with the system creates an eerie and enervating sense of cognitive dissonance. Something is off and dystopian.

People joke that at restaurants, women visit the restroom in pairs. Wherever those impulses originate, we should double down on them when it comes to the healthcare system. Depending on where you are in your life, you can find a friend or be one, and there are smart and strategic ways to go about it that can make a marked difference. While doctors, employees, hospital administrators, and entrepreneurs can all play a role in dismantling the grip that greed has on our healthcare system—and I believe necessity will eventually force this result—women, the gatherers, givers, culture keepers, and role models, can start the necessary revolution, one pair of confidantes at a time. Walking together when we're filled with fear or when we feel disenfranchised is so much better than walking alone. It can change the journey.

TIPS AND TAKEAWAYS

READING LIST

There are important books about greed in American health-care that I recommend, a couple of which I have referenced in this chapter. Each offers compelling information that every informed medical consumer should know.

Never Pay the First Bill: And Other Ways to Fight the Health Care System and Win by Marshall Allen

An American Sickness: How Healthcare Became Big Business and How You Can Take It Back by Elisabeth Rosenthal

The Price We Pay: What Broke American Health Care and How to Fix It by Marty Makary

We've Got You Covered: Rebooting American Health Care by Liran Einav and Amy Finkelstein

The Healing of America: A Global Quest for Better, Cheaper, and Fairer Health Care by T. R. Reid

Deadly Spin: An Insurance Company Insider Speaks Out on How Corporate PR Is Killing Health Care and Deceiving Americans by Wendell Potter

❰ 11 ❱

The Safety Net

IN OVER TWENTY-FIVE years of working with women with
breast and ovarian cancer as a volunteer workplace and patient
advocate, I have likely gotten to speak with well over a thousand human beings in crisis. While many of the questions and
challenges that they had fell into patterns, I also note that each
person and situation was totally distinct. On the person side,
that's in keeping with my philosophy and favorite aphorism,
"Always remember that you are absolutely unique. Just like
everyone else,"[1] and I believe it with my whole soul. On the
situation side, however, this uniqueness can only be called baf-
fling. If every time a person interfaces with the medical system
they must walk through an idiosyncratic labyrinth to get the
care they need and access the benefits they have earned, what
have we got? The most inefficient system imaginable, that's
what. Based on the experiences of the many women I have
worked with, I can attest not only to this inefficiency but also
to the maddening level of stress and nearly intolerable level
of chaos that it causes people who are already in crisis. I have
seen that women bear this chaos disproportionately, especially

women of color. The women struggling in this system are daughters, sisters, mothers, wives, partners, and friends.

One day, I got a call from Bay Area Cancer Connections telling me that they had a client for me to talk to, a woman with an ovarian cancer recurrence who was desperate to get our local teaching hospital to accept her Medicare so that she could get the treatment she needed quickly from the best providers available. In other words, what anyone deserves. Her other choice was to wait for treatment at a county hospital that would take her Medicare but did not have the resources to act fast. She'd been trying to get what she needed for months already, and time was obviously of the essence. When I called her, I could not believe the force of nature on the other end of the line. First off, she had a Brooklyn accent, and being a stranger in a strange land myself (a kid born in Queens living in the Silicon Valley), I immediately warmed to her. Then she told me a little bit about herself. The mother of two professional athletes, she was also a creative producer for film and TV, a nonprofit leader, a poet, and a painter. After college, she'd studied languages and art. A talented, beautiful soul and a make-things-happen human. We had an instant connection, the kind you wake up in the morning hoping for. We put our heads together and with much effort and energy made the right phone calls, wrote strategically worded letters and emails, and succeeded in getting her seen and treated, inside of a week, because we both knew every minute counted. We joked that it would be fun to work together again under better circumstances because we had a creative kinship as well as the worldly chops to make moves. But it took many hours of the two of us harnessing all our savvy and experience just to get to what should have been the status quo: immediate action in the face of an aggressive cancer.

In January of 2016, I got this email from her:

Dear Rebecca,

I hope that you feel the love coming through this email. For the first time in a long time you gave me hope that I can get the proper care, I cannot thank you enough.

I am hopeful that I am moving in the right direction to finally get the care needed to breathe, to live.

Please forward me your address, I would like to send you my poetry & art book. I know that we will meet soon but wanted to send anyway. Can't wait to meet you. . .

I received her book soon after with this gorgeous inscription:

May we always keep peace and love in our heart.
Thank you for all that you do and say! —Karen

Karen lived until October of that year. I'm still devastated by the loss of her light here on earth. I feel for her loved ones and will always yearn for the deepening friendship that might have been. Who knows, maybe we really would have worked together in some way on something that we both cared about.

I treasure the book she sent me and the lovely interchange that we had, but I continue to be haunted by how a woman so creative, capable, successful, classy, giving, and spiritual could have found herself on the wrong end of what was nothing short of an American-healthcare-system-induced crisis. Just when she most needed the system to serve her. When I work with someone like Karen, my resolve becomes stronger. I get wild-eyed with the goal of helping every ill woman I can possibly assist. There is something in me that cannot abide the way things are, how they have been for way too long. The history of healthcare in America is damning. We put profits before people, and the problems this causes continue to worsen.

How Did We Get Here?

How did we get to this place? Where so many people in America are one illness away from economic devastation and people cannot access the care they need without overwhelming friction? I have saved this inquiry for the last chapter in this book, though logic might dictate that it should be the first. But getting up close and personal with women who faced impossible choices at an excruciating moment has been simultaneously devastating and energizing. Consequently, I decided to deliver the stories and the tools that readers can use to match the immediacy of their concerns. So that they could open this book and find solace and practical help from the start. I mean to serve readers and every woman I can when she gets sick. To do this as well as possible, I have also become obsessed with understanding how our system has evolved, from its roots to its tentacles.

The Beginning of Our Healthcare System

Here's what I have learned: Around the start of the twentieth century, before the doctors-golf-on-Wednesday jokes, when Big Pharma wasn't even a gleam in an industrialist's eye, there were no health laws. Doctors usually had home offices, and neither they nor hospitals were too worried about a sea of regulation. They made house calls. If you got sick and needed a doctor, you were typically much more worried about missing work and not getting paid than you were about a bill that would sink you. There wasn't much medical technology to speak of and not that many things doctors could do for their patients. It had been only about fifty years since the discovery of basic bacteriology and even fewer years since the first use of the X-ray.[2] Around 1910, drugs were used to attack certain diseases and surgery became something to try for things like tumors and tonsils.[3] It wasn't that complicated.

There were no health insurance policies for some very simple reasons, mostly math-related. The insurance companies could not figure out how to manage the risks because only people who were sick would try to buy coverage. They couldn't figure out how to price policies to make it make sense for them as a business proposition. Incidentally, the derisively named "Obamacare mandate" that we've all heard so much about, which is a provision of what was formally called the Affordable Care Act of 2008, got right to the heart of this matter, providing that people must buy insurance or pay a fine. Risk spreading is the cornerstone of any insurance system. The ACA was designed this way because if you can't find a way to get people to buy policies, you can't spread the risk among the sick and the healthy. That means way more expensive policies. If they are prohibitively expensive, people opt to self-insure instead. More on the political realities and fate of that later, but spoiler, in many states they've stripped the first *A* for *affordable* right out of the ACA.

Back to early twentieth-century America, before the Great Depression. European countries started to institute national health insurance. But here in the US, neither doctors nor the insurance companies were interested.[4]

But regulation of doctors and hospitals started to take root. In 1910 a report known as "The Flexner Report" called for the professionalization of medical schools, things like stricter entrance standards, higher fees, and more state-of-the-art (for the time) facilities.[5] Low and behold, the income and prestige associated with being a doctor increased, and patient costs rose. As more hospitals got built, home care receded because of sterility concerns and general increases in equipment, devices, and staff.

What happened next wasn't a great shock. Groups began to form to negotiate prepaid plans for hospital care to save money. It's the American way. Sometimes it would be a group like teachers and a local hospital. Other times, it would be a group of hospitals in a region. The goal was two-sided: affordable care on one side and steady income for providers on the other. That made sense, especially after the economic devastation of the Great Depression. By 1937 there were twenty-six of these plans nationwide, with six hundred thousand members in total out of a population of 128.8 million.[6] They banded together to form the Blue Cross Network. In a nifty legislative trick, states gave Blue Cross plans nonprofit status and let them skip the rules that applied to commercial insurance companies, things like requirements that they keep big cash reserves.[7] Right around this time, there were some national health insurance proposals being floated, and primary care doctors worried that maybe those, along with the rise of Blue Cross, would prevent them from setting their own fees. So, they formed another plan just for primary care, Blue Shield. Blue Cross and Blue Shield were able to work by focusing on the young, the healthy, and the employed. With those subscribers, they had a shot at keeping costs down and premiums low. When Congress passed the 1935 Social Security Act (considered to be the bulwark of the "safety net"), not a word was written about health insurance. It's not hard to see why, given the economic forces at play. The safety net was never fully safe, even at its inception.

The Workplace Connection

Flash forward to World War II. Prices and wages were being controlled, so how could employers attract qualified employees? Thus began the golden age of what used to be called "benefits" or "perks." The most valuable one of all was health insurance. It still is. The government realized that health insurance was something to be subsidized—through the back door of the taxation system, anyway. What took root was a deduction for the employer, and a thing of great value that was not considered taxable income for the employee. The government created what they call "incentives" for employers to provide health insurance for employees. On its face, that seems like a sane policy. That is, until the costs to insure employees balloon, and you consider who wasn't reaping the benefits. Also, this was well before there was a firm grasp on who was qualified for the benefits. Was the definition of a qualified employee based on the type of employer (a factory, but not a restaurant?), the type of employee (a white, college-educated man who was born in the US, but not a woman of color who was born elsewhere?), the number of hours worked (assuming those hours are "on the books" and part of what people think of as a "legitimate business," and who decides *this*? Hint: it wasn't usually the marginalized employee). So much unforeseen complexity emerged.

Reimbursement

Here's where things started to go off the rails. Blue Cross and Blue Shield devised a method of reimbursement called "cost plus." And it went like this: doctors got paid "reasonable and customary charges" (that they set themselves) and hospitals were reimbursed based on a formula that was a percentage of their actual costs *plus* a percentage of their working/equity capital. This created the skewed incentives. Doctors charged as much as they could—as much as the market would bear—and hospitals pushed hard on their cost-based charges because they were only getting a percentage back. I call this the "funny money" approach. When more commercial insurance companies and government plans were established (Medicare and Medicaid), this was the game, so they had to play it.

It isn't as though politicians didn't realize that this mélange of a payment system was problematic. President Franklin Roosevelt asked Congress to include satisfactory medical care for every American in his 1944 Economic Bill of Rights. Congress did not oblige. President Harry Truman tried again, but the American Medical Association flipped him the bird (nowadays more physicians support it),[8] and Congress called it a communist plot![9]

In the postwar period, healthcare costs began to escalate. Hospital care became much more expensive, medications and vaccines were introduced, and surgeries became more sophisticated. At the same time, the 1960s saw a pronounced rise in new health insurance companies, but the unemployed, underemployed, impoverished, and elderly were going without. Since it was clear that the political will to pass universal healthcare could not be drummed up, Congress had to come up with another plan, and that's how we ended up with Medicare and Medicaid in 1965, to cover the elderly and the poor, respectively.[10] Immediately, these two programs adopted the same broken reimbursement processes, and they were the biggest payers for healthcare services in the country from the moment they were created, triggering an endless cycle of healthcare inflation. Doctors and hospitals keep charging more as reimbursements falter. The prices aren't real. It's a never-ending game of hand over hand.

The Managed Care Phase

I call the next part of this story the *managed care phase*. This is where we learn those acronyms "HMO" (Health Maintenance Organization) and "PPO" (Preferred Provider Organization) that perplex us if we're lucky enough to have the kind of employment that offers us such plans to begin with. The original HMO, Kaiser Permanente, started out as the Kaiser Foundation Health Plan, a prepaid health benefits program for employees who worked in Kaiser shipyards.[11] This model of care delivery has become an efficiency standard bearer, cutting costs by minimizing utilization and shortening hospital stays. That saves money. It's not all bad, and some of my dearest friends have made careers caring deeply for patients despite the "do it in twelve minutes" rules. But saving money was the inciting goal. Then, in 1973, Congress passed the Health Maintenance Organization Act to spur the growth of HMOs, offering them grants and loans to start up and requiring employers with more than twenty-five employees to offer these plans alongside traditional fee-for-service health insurance plans.[12] This law had the intended effect. By 1991, there were over 550 HMOs with over thirty-five million subscribers, compared to only twenty-six HMOs with three million in 1970.[13] Managed care. Cost cutting. It was on.

Medicare and Medicaid Changes

At the same time, Medicare and Medicaid fell into crisis. To keep up with escalating costs they added a giant headache to whatever else might be ailing a patient. In the early eighties, Medicare came out with diagnosis-related groups (DRGs). Basically these were categories of illnesses that were identified for purposes of reimbursing hospitals, under a system known as the prospective payment system. It worked with set rates. For example, for an embolism, we pay "X." Sorry, hospitals and doctors, but that's what you get. The idea was to control costs, but it resulted in hospitals trying, instead, to shift the excess costs to patients.[14] These healthcare plans were for low-income and the elderly. Premiums were subsidized because in most cases, these folks could not afford them! So passing unreimbursed costs *onto them* was a recipe for disaster. Congress had to try again in the early nineties. This time, tying Medicare and Medicaid reimbursements to the cost of resources consumed. This worked, perhaps, a little better, but the system is so complicated that it's hard to say. In many cases now, doctors and hospitals have decided they just won't treat Medicare and Medicaid patients because it's too frustrating and they barely get paid. It's hard to call that a win.

Escalating Costs

The last two decades of the twentieth century saw costs rise exponentially. This was partially due to all the new and expensive technology being developed, but also because there were cutbacks to the incentives for HMOs. As opposed to overseas, where universal healthcare systems were successful in keeping a lid on drug costs, the price of medications in America were inflated because of this crazy third-party payer system and the fact that here most Big Pharma research and development costs get passed on to the consumer. During the Clinton administration, then First Lady Hillary Clinton worked with then director of the Office of Management and Budget, Leon Panetta, on a "managed competition" idea that was another angle on universal coverage, but it died a political death.[15] Due to pressure from consumers and employers, even managed care plans began to push back on draconian cost-cutting such as end-of-life care limits and physician choice.

The Affordable Care Act

By the time President Obama passed the Affordable Care Act in 2010, it was clear that universal healthcare was as politically elusive as ever. The ACA was complicated and ambitious, amending a bevy of existing laws and clocking in at over a thousand pages. Implementation was a feat, but the bottom line is that so far it has added more than thirty-one million people to the ranks of the insured and withstood three Supreme Court challenges to date. The first phase of the law requires people to be insured or pay a penalty, expands Medicaid, blocks insurers from denying anyone coverage due to preexisting conditions, requires large employers to provide coverage, and establishes reimbursement plans based on patient outcomes as opposed to volume of services provided. These are all big steps that were implemented in 2010. The following year, more aspects of the law became effective: kids stay on their parents' insurance until age twenty-six, plans must cover preventive care, lifetime caps on coverage are eliminated, and consumers receive rebates if insurers spend too much on advertising and too little on quality of care. By 2012, a Supreme Court case upheld the penalty on people who didn't buy health insurance, but states were allowed to choose whether to expand Medicaid. Meaning that poor people in red states—at least initially—wouldn't benefit. The law rolled out further. By 2013 and 2014, online marketplaces for policies known as state exchanges were opening. From 2010 through the first nine months of 2015, the uninsured rate fell by more than 40 percent. With Donald Trump's 2016 election, this progress began to unravel. House Republicans tried to repeal the ACA. They failed, but Congress eliminated the penalty for not having health insurance. Meaning costs would go up because there wouldn't be enough healthy buyers in the pool (as of this writing, premium price increases have already outpaced the cost of living). More legal challenges ensued, but the ACA, though hobbled, survived the Trump administration.[16] For now, we are left with something complicated that isn't particularly affordable after all. At least individuals who don't have employer-provided coverage can buy coverage without the fear that a preexisting condition will leave them in a health crisis boat without a health insurance paddle—but those plans are far from affordable for most.

None other than the US Government has gone on record to warn citizens about how expensive healthcare is and how important it is for people to find coverage. The healthcare.gov website notes in 2023 that a broken leg can run $7500, three days in a hospital averages $30,000, and "comprehensive cancer care can cost hundreds of thousands of dollars."[17] The site explicitly states that health coverage can protect people from "high, unexpected costs like these."[18] Yet, finding such coverage is still a maze. It is not categorically affordable, and even in cases where a woman is covered, she can still find herself in debt or facing bankruptcy due to an illness. Since 2006, Massachusetts has provided state-level universal healthcare for its citizens. In fact, their laws inspired the ACA on the national level. In 2024, all low-income adults will be eligible for free health coverage in California. But universal healthcare at the state level is a hard nut to crack because the expense is so significant. Blue states like California and Vermont have made legislative attempts, as have "purple" states like Colorado, but they have failed (or in the case of Vermont, it passed but was shelved).[19] Colorado, Nevada, and Washington have been able to pass a "public option," but it is opt-in only, as opposed to universal. Like many other hot-button political issues, there is no national consensus, and a state-by-state approach is far less effective than a national one from an implementation standpoint.[20]

The takeaway is that no matter who you are, no matter your coverage or employment status, if you find yourself with cancer or other serious diagnosis, you will need to get your ducks in a row to understand what will and won't be covered and how you're going to manage your work life. This is true for everyone, but it is particularly the case when it comes to women.

There Are Holes in Our Safety Net, But Advocacy Can Help

The system failed my friend Karen, may she rest in power and beauty. She worked her whole life and paid into the so-called safety net. It did not keep her safe. The failure of the healthcare system is nothing short of a failure of the social contract.

Karen eventually got that care she sought, but we had to fight
for it after considerable delay. I have often wondered if getting
her help sooner might have made the difference or at least
given her more time. This is the hardest part of doing this
work.

Every woman who gets sick deserves to be cared for and
cradled within a functional safety net. Until we get to a better
place in this country, all women with cancer or other serious
illness must fight for their right to heal and thrive. I am fighting alongside them because I have seen that having an advocate who can anticipate problems, follow up on paperwork
and phone calls, ask pertinent questions about treatments and
protocols, explore options for employment extension, and
secure insurance coverage and income replacement can make
a difference. As can fair-minded, compassionate, and radical
listening.

Not every woman I have worked with gets better. But
I hope that the journeys of those who did not were better
because of how we communicated and collaborated. A woman
with a terminal illness is sentient, worthy and alive, no less so
than someone who believes they have countless years ahead of
them. I had a call with a woman recently who told me that
a specialist had told her he did not want to pursue further
treatment because of the number of spots on her PET Scan.
If there had been fewer, he'd have proceeded, he told her, but
according to the scan, he deemed her a "bad bet." I am not a
doctor, and I do not know what the right medical or financial

decision was in that situation. But I am a professional communicator, and I do know that no woman should be dehumanized and treated like a statistic at such an excruciating moment. Words matter. Respect matters. Our system has created this dynamic, and our compassion is being rationed along with our limited resources. Supporting women, connecting, and caring are all good bets to me.

Conclusion
We Can Make This Better for Women

IT ISN'T HARD to find groups of people who rally around a woman they know who is experiencing a health challenge. Most people are decent, and many are remarkably generous. But our country has never amassed the political will to take care of our sick outside of the microcosms we build for ourselves. We have never, as a republic, decided that we view healthcare as a fundamental right available to all. Healthcare is not part of our safety net. It is not within our definition of "life, liberty, and the pursuit of happiness." This is not a partisan issue, though it might appear so on the surface. As soon as you or a woman you love needs care or medication and is unable to get it, this is about you, whether you're politically red, blue, purple, or polka-dotted.

Women bear the brunt, particularly low-income women and women of color. We have normalized this when we should normalize a more humane, holistic notion of how to take care of ourselves, our bodies, and our loved ones. I had a wonderful conversation with social worker, educator, and women's health nonprofit leader, Amy Goldsbury, on this topic. As a young mother, Amy was diagnosed with stage 4 colon cancer, which required surgery and debilitating treatments. Amy worried that her son was too young to remember her if she didn't make it. It was intense. With extraordinary support from her friends, family, and forward-thinking employer and colleagues, Amy triumphed. People in the school district she worked at donated their sick days so she could take time off for treatment. While I believe that employers and governments can come up with more generous sick leave plans, possibly even more practical and disease-specific, I nonetheless laud the selflessness of Amy's coworkers. Her mother took a leave of absence from work to help her care for her son. Her former soccer team circled around her. She had excellent health insurance, caring doctors, and a supportive spouse. All of this strengthened her for her battle. She knows people who had the identical diagnosis who were not so lucky. I thought Amy was the perfect person to ask about how we can make this system work better for women because she was the recipient of so much well-deserved and creatively delivered goodness. She also spent six years working at a cancer support organization after her illness, so her thoughts come from her own experience and the many things she learned helping other people through their cancer journeys.

The first thing Amy noted is that women handle so much. They run their homes even when they work outside of them. From her own experience, she said, we've got to form what she calls circles of goodness around women when they get sick, because in those moments, they cannot handle everything. Amy calls for a culture where it is okay for women to ask for help and be willing to accept it. She believes that this kind of thinking must extend to the workplace, as do I. We should all accept that illness happens often. It's a human experience, not an opportunity for othering. As Amy puts it, "It's not unique to just certain families. Nearly every family is touched by cancer or another serious illness."

Amy's point is that it shouldn't be out of the ordinary for employers to be flexible with scheduling and give sick employees and caregivers time off. As she says, "We have to be able to look after each other." At her job at a school district, Amy oversaw discipline, and teachers would send her referrals to work with students who were having behavioral problems. Even though she was out, colleagues sent reports along to keep Amy in the loop, but with them were cards saying simple things like "we're missing you" and "we're thinking about you." It meant so much to her to be acknowledged. Amy notes that generally in US culture, "we do not do illness well." She's right. We're uncomfortable and we tend to freeze. We often cut people out unwittingly—sick people who need to be accompanied as they trudge through—because we don't know what to say.

Amy learned from her own experiences and brought them to the programming she did in her job at Cancer CARE-point, a cancer organization in San Jose, California. One of her goals was to teach better communication. Amy remembers "a parent who was going through breast cancer shared that her ten-year-old son expressed confusion about why people were bringing food to the house. He told his mom that he thought her sickness must be bad if they couldn't even cook dinner themselves. That's what went on in his little ten-year-old brain. And nobody explained it to him and said that people were just trying to find some way to help."[1] Through the eyes of a child, this is a powerful illustration of discomfort borne of fear. People say too much or too little. They drop off the food and go because it's awkward. Children, perhaps our keenest and most honest observers, feel it for all of us.

Amy points out that it isn't only friends, community members, children, and caregivers who are uncomfortable when a woman gets sick. Unease with disease hits the workplace too. She cites a moment during her journey when she attended a retirement party in her district for an administrator, who "acknowledged several up-and-coming young professionals who were there," but did not mention her, though she was similarly situated. Amy knows it wasn't ill will, but it highlights the psychosocial issues that abound when a woman gets sick.

She also feels that so much of the support available to women comes only in a medical environment, "in a clinical way." The day-to-day interactions can improve in the home, the health space, and the workplace. The only way to set the stage for the better is to raise awareness, tell the stories, and shine light on the human issues. It also takes listening. Because while serious illness happens to many women, each faces a unique situation, and they all deserve individualized attention and support. Serious illness is seismic; it shakes women's lives.

When they are treated with humanity and met with enlightened communication, it makes an enormous difference. That's what Amy found, and she has paid it forward. These cultural shifts feel doable. It's about education and thoughtful communication.

Amy believes that women deserve to be heard and fully seen when sick for a host of moral reasons, but also because they are usually caregivers. She worries most for socioeconomically disadvantaged women and women of color based on her experiences in supporting others and seeing that these groups tend to have fewer systemic options they can rely upon. They take care of others, but few resources are devoted to taking care of them. Amy says, "We know that women of color are not getting the same care as white women. There are things that can be done, like free wig banks and gift cards, but at the end of the day, all women deserve the best possible care and that is not happening." I'm with Amy. Every woman is somebody's daughter. More efforts to level the playing field are needed, and health equity must begin at the institutional level. We have to stand up for this at all levels, federal, state, and local.

The last aspect of my incredible conversation with Amy centered around survivorship. She designed and led eight-week workshops for survivors because she knew that leaving "patient land" and reintegrating has its own set of issues. The majority of the participants were women, and Amy described guiding them through the beautiful and scary process of transitioning from patient to survivor. In these workshops women would reflect on their lives pre-cancer and the work they did, how they were burning themselves out, how they were everything to every person. Through the weeks, the women began to reevaluate and ask themselves, "How do I want to move forward and still take care of myself? Because I've had this huge scare, so I really want to prioritize my health."

But this wasn't always so simple. For many women, this meant thinking of a job change, bringing on questions of financial security, health insurance, and such. Amy says that she and her husband have chosen or not taken jobs to make sure that the health insurance offered would allow her to keep her team of doctors. I wish that every woman who survives an illness could benefit from a workshop like Amy's, and perhaps these are the kinds of changes to our current system that are possible. I've been in contact with social workers at various organizations across the country and have learned that workshops and programming around survivorship are becoming more common, so there is reason to hope on this front.

As Amy's example shows, women who get sick often turn into passionate advocates for others. As part of your health journey, perhaps during your treatments, or maybe as a healing victory lap, you can use your voice, energy, and resources to make things better not only for yourself but for other women who are fighting illness, either in the health space or the workplace. You can also encourage your friends and family to do this as a way of honoring your journey.

This is how communities form and positive change happens. There is no one way to take action, and you and your team can find a way to do something productive that suits your values.

One possibility is to give back and volunteer at a local women's health center. Some of the longest-standing and most dedicated volunteers at Bay Area Cancer Connections, where I've served for over twenty-five years, started out as clients. Like my dear friend Karlette Warner, the original ace hotliner, who has been there on the front lines helping women who called in with questions and challenges for decades. Supporting an organization that has given you help and information when you needed it is a fantastic way to make change and make something good out of the challenges you're facing. Additionally, you can first look for and then run support groups at your employer for other women as they deal with illness. These groups help women navigate the complexities that arise, but they also become keys to making things work for one another. For example, women often band together and create meal preparation teams, form sick leave banks, and design other ways for team members to help each other through illness. Beyond these grassroots ideas, there are ways to connect and volunteer with disease-specific research organizations and participate in walks, runs, and other fundraisers that can be part of your wellness routine. Connecting with groups like this can help you, and it can also give you connection and purpose, both vital to your overall well-being.

Working with brave women as they fight illness sometimes takes my breath away. It's an honor to walk a path with
a person who has the clarity to tell the truth, apply her gifts,
and think about making things better for others as she treads
a tough path herself. So often I have found that women who
could retreat into a cocoon instead choose to make an impact.
Life means more when you're fighting for it daily. Nobody
exemplified this more than my friend Vicky Michelis, and I
am certain she is resting in both peace and power.

Here's how we met: it was 2013, and I was a presenter
at a Bay Area Cancer Connections annual conference at the
Oracle Conference Center in Redwood Shores, California.
Though I adore working closely with individuals and small
groups, public speaking isn't my natural jam. I was nervous
to be in such a grand space and on the ticket with so many
cancer care experts. I wanted so much to deliver something
of value to the conference attendees, a group of earnest information and fellowship seekers. I wanted to empower them in
an electric way. But I was there to talk about issues women
battling illness face in the workplace and the health space,
from insurance to leaves of absence to how to communicate
with doctors. I've always been sensitive about how dry these
topics seem. Levity is a stretch. So, I focused on bringing my
A game for the room full of participants. After laying out a
dense array of information peppered with self-deprecating
jokes about the stuff nobody really wants to know unless they
must, I tried to engage the crowd in some fact-patterns. Not

in a scary law school way, but more folksy, playful and relatable. My point was to get creative thinking and collaboration going, but also to be interactive and hopefully interesting and thought-provoking. Though I clutched at my plastic-covered name tag hanging on the lanyard anxiously, I was thrilled to see that the exercise was working. The audience was responsive and witty and cared about the hypotheticals that I presented, based, as they were, on real people. I caught us having some fun together as we creatively problem-solved.

When the session ended, women filed out, warming me with their hugs, thanks, and lovely comments. I couldn't imagine feeling better about an experience. And then it was elevated. A lovely, tall woman with piercing eyes waited until everyone else left to introduce herself. Her name tag said *Vicky Michelis*. She extended her hand and introduced herself, and we struck up a conversation. Wow, was she articulate and energized. She shared that she had been battling ovarian cancer and was in remission. She wanted to talk to me about her plans to start an ovarian cancer awareness organization to help women learn more about signs and symptoms, to advocate for the development of early detection tests, and to support women going through what she had been through.

"I really enjoyed your presentation, and you said you're a former lawyer." She paused and smiled. "I couldn't help but wonder if you might know about 501(c)(3) formation . . ."

I laughed. Because I recognized her can-do spirit immediately. This was a woman who saw possibility and figured out to make things happen. I later found out she'd worked in logistics for a major tech company. That checked out. We agreed to a brainstorming coffee. I offered all the help I could, and I'm still not sure she needed me because nothing was going to stop her. We emailed back and forth, and I gladly gave advice and support. She founded Teal's Real, a fabulous organization devoted to educating women about developments in ovarian cancer. She teamed up with motorcycle groups riding across the state to raise money for prostate cancer and convinced them to work for ovarian cancer as well and organized 5k foot race fundraisers and support groups. Everyone in the local cancer community knew Vicky because she was so generous, broad-minded, capable, creative, and kind. I loved being her friend and supporter.

When she called me a few years later to tell me about her recurrence, she was hopeful and positive. That's how she was, even in the face of some truly absurd insurance denials for treatments and medications at her longtime healthcare provider. We worked together on straightening things out. Her sense of humor and equanimity were amazing to behold. I was fit to be tied and cursing like a sailor, and she shrugged it off as bureaucracy that we'd beat together. She said she knew I'd bust through the wall because she knew me. I wish with all my heart that she had been the beneficiary of a medical breakthrough on top of the coverage and care that should have been a given. Nobody fought harder for progress for other women and nobody deserved a miracle more. She passed in 2020, leaving a community of friends, colleagues, and admirers. I ran a virtual 5k in her honor in the middle of the pandemic, smile-crying the whole time. I still have my teal rubber bracelet.

While I had no doubt that Vicky and her example of activism and dedication to the wellness of others would live in my heart always, I didn't expect what happened next. When someone close to me heard I was working on this book, he connected me to Amy Goldsbury, the wonderful woman I wrote about earlier in this section. Amy and I talked about the way cancer changes people. How small talk means less and action means more. And then she said, "Like my friend Vicky." My eyes welled up. I knew immediately that she was talking about my Vicky. Our Vicky. My new friend Amy went on to tell me something unforgettable, but also unsurprising. Vicky left fellow cancer survivors bequests in her last will and testament. Generous ones. They came with letters that said things like "Please use this for a family vacation. You deserve that." Each letter included the ask that one thousand dollars be paid forward. Vicky asked her beneficiaries to do things like give hardworking waitresses one hundred-dollar tips or help out a neighbor in need, no questions asked. She also asked all her beneficiaries to create a private online group so they could share and inspire one another with stories about how they'd used the money. The group brainstormed together about how they could continue to spread that spirit around.

Amy's connection to Vicky nearly knocked me over. A friend, activist, cancer warrior, and exemplary human being came back to me. Vicky's goodness, grace, and light are renewable and present in those she touched. If people could be more like Vicky, if they could care about all women, not only their own, just imagine.

You've heard it said: "Health is wealth." I have learned, up close and repeatedly, that this truism can't be overstated. Just ask any woman who is on a health journey what she wishes for most. Women and all people deserve the best chance to be well that our society can provide. It stands to reason that health equity should be among the most pressing social issues.

The complexity of our healthcare system can be enervating. And the way we are served information in today's digital world can sometimes make us feel hopeless, hence the newfangled word *doomscrolling*. But the gender health equity movement has made concrete progress. The Center for Disease Control and the National Institute of Health have made serious investments in bridging the gaps in research, diagnosis, and treatment of women's diseases.[2] Major nonprofits like the American Heart Association have committed to the importance of women's health as well.[3] American businesses have begun to see the writing on the wall. Women's health initiatives are being pursued by major stakeholders because they make economic sense. Startups devoted to women's health improvements are cropping up and attracting robust financing, and books are being published on the subject more than ever before.

When I started this work all those years ago, I felt like a naive do-gooder trying to save women's bodies from a sinking ship. Now, despite changing legal and political winds, I believe women's health is having a moment that will turn into a season and solidify into a cultural shift. To honor the memory of women I've worked with who did not win their battles and help along the healing journeys of those who have been more fortunate, I will stay the course. I hope to share useful information and stories that illustrate what's possible with as many women as I can. It is the work of my lifetime. While our system is surely flawed, even within its cracked walls there is room to make things better for women when they face serious illnesses. Count me in for the long haul. I'll walk with you.

ACKNOWLEDGMENTS

I HAVE ENDLESS gratitude for the people who have helped me get this book out into the world, who saw my purpose and gave me their time, attention, and support.

I want to celebrate my agent extraordinaire, Don Pape. He's full of goodness and intelligence. A champion of writers. A supporter of women and girls and an almost impossibly nice guy. But don't let that fool you. He's an expert literary matchmaker who sees the possible. I used to write contracts for a living, and I'd never want anyone but Don to help me make mine because we share vision and purpose, and that means the world to me.

Through Don's expertise, I met Lisa Kloskin and the amazing team at Broadleaf Books. Lisa is a most insightful, bright, and committed editor (she'd probably strike "most" in that sentence and change the "a" to "an," and normally I might, too, but my feelings are superlative). Her ideas and input made this a better book. Lisa's deep knowledge, fine taste, and her compassion to know when to go deeper into a story helped me get more out of mine.

Dr. Lynn Taylor is my oldest friend. Our bond of over fifty years started out like a lightning bolt and has never waned. Regardless of where we are, we are always aligned.

Her guidance and depth are all over this book. She's a healer's healer. A person of commitment and integrity. I am truly fortunate to be part of her life, and I treasure her.

Dr. Jeremy Boal has been my dear friend and confidant since we were kids. I've never known a more thoughtful, devoted, big-thinking doctor or a kinder, more amazing companion through a system that leaves so many alone. He's helped me connect patients I care about with doctors who can truly help them more times than I can count, and a few of those stories are in this book. He's honest, brave, and virtuous. He blesses every life he touches, starting with mine.

Dr. Kristina Austin is one of my greatest champions, a nearest-and-dearest and a doctor who puts patients first, regardless of what the system throws her way. She's a fierce, quiet leader and a defender of what's right. Currently, Dr. Austin teaches the next generation of doctors, and this fills me with hope, because if they care even half as much as she does, we might just be all right.

Dr. Christie Coleman was my friend first. Then, when I needed her, she became my doctor. At a dark and scary moment, she filled my heart with light the way only a badass saver of women's and babies' lives can.

Dr. Lynn Smolik is the doctor I choose to take care of me. She knows who I am, understands my risks and sensitivities, and has never failed to be there for me with excellent care and practically perfect communication.

Dr. Cherie Futerman is the epitome of excellence and integrity. She gives women her absolute best and is on a mission to detect cancer as early as possible and save lives. I am so lucky to be her patient and her friend.

Dr. Susan Lewis is a consummate professional who gives her all to keeping women active and healthy. She treats her patients like family, follows up with sincere concern, and always fits people in when they need to be seen. I thought it was just me, but it is her!

Dr. Stacey Budin, I don't think I can ever thank you enough for your wisdom, kindness and support. But I will keep trying!

Pamela Weiss is a brilliant and generous collaborator. Thank you for caring so much, supporting my work with your signature oomph, giving me guidance, storytelling purpose, and a view of the bigger picture. And, of course, thank you for your trust and confidence. Working with you at lifting up women's stories is an honor and a joy.

Debra Landwehr Engle, you know what this work means to me. Thank you for caring so much and guiding me. Julie Cantrell, I respect you as a writer and teacher and deeply appreciate your support. Stephanie Raffelock, the questions we've posed and the structures we've structured! Laura Rhodes Levin, we did some things! Jill Sherer Murray, cousin, your savvy mind, creative practicality, and humor have fueled me. Teresa Drosselmeyer, you generously read and commented on some early drafts and I'm so grateful. Sarah Stall, I'm so thrilled to word nerd with you, thank you. Babs Cheung, woman, you are so smart and delightful to know, I'd let you read my mother's chart, I swear. Robin Bell Nobles, your care, kindness and way of being fills my heart. Michelle Schuman, you are a badass human, and you've inspired me to be better and do what I can to make a dent, no matter how colossal the problem. Constance Nicole Frierson, your trust, confidence, bravery, kindness, and loyalty have sustained me. Frances Denny, thank you for sharing your beautiful world with me.

Kim, Rachel, Alison, and Julia Sommer are my girls! Having this team of power women in my corner has been like a protein shake at mile twenty-one. Alice Hom, my first California friend. Cristina and Sara Vitale, you know.

Allan Heinberg has been part of my firmament since 1985. He's my go-to for how to tell a story and has taught me so much about how to love and how to communicate. Ours is a forty-years-and-counting conversation about what makes our hearts sing. He can hold the melody or bring the harmony. Shelley Onderdonk started out as a college friend and roommate, but became a colleague, supporter, and collaborator. I adore and respect her and the way she cares about the health and wellness of all living things. Tracy Lassin Cappas, Julie Malork Schindler, Dr. Jennifer Robohm, I love each of you for always.

Stefanie Harris is the one I got through the formative years with and she's never let me down. Since seventh grade. Leslie Lefkowitz and Tracey Stein West, you two mean so much to me. You rescued a nerd's nerd from the grade below and gave me a lifetime of friendship, love, goodness, and precious memories. Each of you has always stood for me and I will always stand for you.

Lisa Otsuka, everyone has a favorite English teacher and you are mine. You're the best reader, the most ardent supporter, and the two of all twos on the Enneagram. You make me feel seen and known.

Alisa Figueroa is a warrior for what's right. She stands for honesty, openness, and unconditional love. Thank you, my friend. Amy Goldsbury is a generous giant in the world. Amy, thank you so much for sharing your experiences and wisdom.

My friends from Bay Area Cancer Connections, Rina Bello, Amy Moody, Sonia Sifuentes, Karlette Warner, Colleen Carvahlo, and Erika Bell, you've done so much to support my work, and I don't know how to thank you for the fellowship and common purpose. Thank you for introducing me to my friend and colleague, Sarah McDonald. Sarah, you inspire me.

I'm so lucky and grateful to know an amazing group of book professionals. The following people gave their time generously and offered me excellent advice about how to get through the publishing process, and I'm thankful: Lisa Tener, Brooke Warner, Laura Mazer, Renee Fountain, Cecilia Lyra, and Joelle Hahn.

Molly Antos and Dana Smith, are you kidding me? I couldn't be luckier than to know such amazing women, much less work with you more than once.

Emma Phelps, your energy, time, and helpful research mean the world to me, as does your belief in this work.

To my Park Slope, Brooklyn, family Jack Nayer, Josephine Ho, and Cynthia Lane. This book was born on Garfield Place and that's where I finished it too. You are all so special to me.

Christine Butler! Not everyone is so lucky to have a dear friend who happens to be an excellent professional photographer. You made the headshot process feel more like a safe safari on a beautiful day. I thank you so much for sharing your talent and heart with me. Phenomenal writer and thinker Amy Herman, I am wowed and honored by your support.

Sarah Elizabeth Greer, your way of seeing a story has changed my brain. You helped me figure out how to make this work accessible, meaningful, and helpful—a book people might read. You spent time listening and creatively coached me to unfold something true and painful yet lace it with the right balance of hope and joy. Nobody could have guided me better or with more profound kindness, generosity, and honesty. I adore you.

I have an incredible family. My mother, Linda Ackerman, is beyond bright, talented, tasteful, sassy, loving, insightful, and just so very beautiful that I can't believe she's mine. My father, I could write a whole book about this guy, but in addition to being the most adorable, wise and generous person on earth, he taught me how to live a life of purpose and perspective. The support that this power couple has given me could never be exaggerated. They are my everything and with good reason. My siblings, David and Dan Ackerman and Ellen Pollack, are more than just my first friends. They are leaders, givers, thinkers, and excellent humans. Thanks, Mom and Dad, for each of them! I adore my aunt Betty Clarick, my aunt Nancy Cook-Dubin and my uncle and aunt Jeffrey and Judy Cook. Each of them makes me feel so loved and known. Cousins! I have the best! Rennie, Jon, Jane, Greg, Rob, and Alison—Nana would be so proud of all of you! Jesse, Noah, Elisa, Laura, and Dan—Bub and Zayde adored you all for reasons I understand. Amy and Merilee Newman, I'm looking at you! Kate Shepherd! Stephanie and Debra Bloom, Yvette Ackerman and Naomi Shapiro, my amazing sisters-in-law, you are all so important to me. Ken Bloom, you are a brother to me. Frank Bloom, thank you. Ali, Rachel, Matt, Jessica, Miriam, Nate, Josh, Elijah, Rosie, Zach, Allie, and Zoe—you all fill my heart with hope and love.

I mention the names of departed family members because they are with me every day, right behind my eyes. I now know that love lasts beyond a lifetime. Rose Silinsky Cook, J. Philip Cook, Beatrice Mendelsohn Ackerman, Sydney Ackerman, Suzanne Shepherd, Laurence Cook-Dubin, Sydney Ackerman Jr., Tema Ackerman, Donald Clarick, Esther Cook Weiner, Jacqui Morgan, Thelma Newman and Lou Newman, Scott Bloom and Sheila Bloom. Your memories are a blessing and a clarion call.

My husband, Jeff, has been by my side through every minute of this journey since 1L, supporting me with his signature smarts, generosity, integrity, sensitivity, patience, and unconditional love. Thank you for giving me the thumbs-up so I could boldly go where I felt I was needed. You always understood what it was about for me and in the wider world. You're the very best partner, father, and man. I love you.

My daughters, Samantha and Olivia, have given me a renewed sense of who I want to be and are my greatest teachers. Sam, you're a brilliant storyteller, deep thinker, and get-it-done-right human. Your talent, wit, and beauty are off the page, yet your astonishing kindness knocks me out even more. Olivia, your prodigious talent, inimitable style, and strength blow my mind, as does your loyalty and unwavering goodness. I am amazed by your insight always. Jack Coolbaugh and John Gardner, thank you for loving them. I'm right there with you!

Above all, I thank the many women who have honored me with their trust during their health journeys. I am better for having known each of you. Thank you so very much.

R.B.

NOTES

Chapter 1: Set Yourself Up for Support

1. US Census Bureau, "Census Bureau Releases New Estimates on America's Families and Living Arrangements," Census.gov, November 30, 2021, https://www.census.gov/newsroom/press-releases/2021/families-and-living-arrangements.html.

2. Emine Saner, "The Breakup Guru Who Invented Conscious Uncoupling: 'I Understand the Backlash,'" *The Guardian*, April 22, 2018, https://www.theguardian.com/lifeandstyle/2018/apr/22/the-breakup-guru-who-invented-conscious-uncoupling-i-understand-the-backlash.

3. Bridget Lavelle and Pamela J. Smock, "Divorce and Women's Risk of Health Insurance Loss," *Journal of Health and Social Behavior* 53, no. 4 (November 12, 2012): 413–31, https://doi.org/10.1177/0022146512465758.

4. US Census Bureau, "Census Bureau Releases New Estimates on America's Families and Living Arrangements."

5. Robin Bleiweis, Diana Boesch, and Alexandra Cawthorne Gaines, "The Basic Facts About Women in Poverty," *American Progress*, August 3, 2022, https://www.americanprogress.org/article/basic-facts-women-poverty/.

6. Ehrenreich, Barbara. *Nickel and Dimed: On (Not) Getting By in America*. Picador, 2011.

7. Sharon R. Johnson et al., "Cancer, Employment, and American Indians: A Participatory Action Research Pilot Study," *Rehabilitation Counseling Bulletin* 54, no. 3 (September 2, 2010): 175–80, https://doi.org/10.1177/0034355210380143.

8. Victoria S. Blinder and Franceca M. Gany, "Impact of Cancer on Employment," *Journal of Clinical Oncology* 38, no. 4 (February 1, 2020): 302–9, https://doi.org/10.1200/jco.19.01856.

9. Gretchen Borchelt, "The Impact Poverty Has on Women's Health," *Human Rights Magazine*, 43:3, https://www.americanbar.org/groups/crsj/publications/human_rights_magazine_home/the-state-of-healthcare-in-the-united-states/poverty-on-womens-health/.

10. Borchelt, "The Impact Poverty Has."

11. Jennifer Tolbert, Patrick Drake, and Anthony Damico, "Key Facts About the Uninsured Population," KFF, December 18, 2023, https://www.kff.org/uninsured/issue-brief/key-facts-about-the-uninsured-population/.

12. Tolbert et al., "Key Facts."

13. "Women's Health Insurance Coverage," KFF, February 6, 2024, https://www.kff.org/womens-health-policy/fact-sheet/womens-health-insurance-coverage/.

14. Borchelt, "The Impact Poverty Has."

Chapter 2: What Kind of Help to Ask For

1. Office for Civil Rights, "The HIPAA Privacy Rule," HHS.gov, July 22, 2024, https://www.hhs.gov/hipaa/for-professionals/privacy/index.html.

2. Tracy Kidder, *Mountains Beyond Mountains: The Quest of Dr. Paul Farmer, a Man Who Would Cure the World* (New York: Random House Trade Paperbacks, 2004).
3. "The Myth of Female Hysteria and Health Disparities Among Women," RTI, May 9, 2018, https://www.rti.org/insights/myth-female-hysteria-and-health-disparities-among-women.

Chapter 4: Taming the Health Insurance Beast

1. "Stress About Health Insurance Costs Reported by Majority of Americans, APA Stress in America Survey Reveals," *APA*, January 24, 2018, https://www.apa.org/news/press/releases/2018/01/insurance-costs#:~:text=WASHINGTON%20%E2%80%94%20Two%2Dthirds%20of%20U.S.,Americans%20at%20all%20income%20levels.
2. Tori DeAngelis, "Rising Health Care Costs and Access to Care Are Major Stressors—Especially for Women and Hispanic Americans," https://www.apa.org, n.d., https://www.apa.org/monitor/2023/06/women-hispanics-stress-health-care-costs.
3. In many cases, the Consolidated Omnibus Budget Reconciliation Act of 1985 (COBRA) will be a smart move, though it is often expensive. COBRA requires an employer to offer an employee who has experienced certain qualifying events continued coverage under the employer's group health plan at the employee's cost for a period of up to thirty-six months. Qualifying events include the covered employee leaving or losing their job

or reducing work hours, the covered employee enrolling in Medicare, divorce from or the death of a covered employee, or aging out of one's parents' policy when turning twenty-six years old.

Chapter 5: Even If You Have Insurance, Stay Prepared

1. Lunna Lopes et al., "Health Care Debt in the US: The Broad Consequences of Medical and Dental Bills," KFF, February 13, 2024, https://www.kff.org/health-costs/report/kff-health-care-debt-survey/.
2. David U. Himmelstein et al., "Medical Bankruptcy: Still Common Despite the Affordable Care Act," *American Journal of Public Health* 109, no. 3 (March 1, 2019): 431–33, https://doi.org/10.2105/ajph.2018.304901.
3. "Millennials Rack up the Most Medical Debt, and More Frequently," *PBS News*, July 26, 2018, https://www.pbs.org/newshour/health/millennials-rack-up-the-most-medical-debt-and-more-frequently.
4. Michael Sainato, "'I Live on the Street Now': How Americans Fall Into Medical Bankruptcy," *The Guardian*, January 6, 2021, https://www.theguardian.com/us-news/2019/nov/14/health-insurance-medical-bankruptcy-debt.
5. Noam Levey, "Medical Debt Upended Their Lives. Here's What It Took From Them," *NPR*, December 21, 2022, https://www.npr.org/sections/health-shots/2022/06/16/1104969627/medical-debt-upended-.

Chapter 6: Access to Advice, Diagnostics, and Treatment

1. "Across Diseases, Women Are Diagnosed Later Than Men," *ScienceDaily*, March 19, 2019, https://www.sciencedaily. com/releases/2019/03/190311103059.htm.
2. *Harvard Health Blog,* October 9, 2017, https://www. health.harvard.edu/blog/women-and-pain-disparities-in-experience-and-treatment-2017100912562.
3. Jayne Leonard, "Gender Bias in Medical Diagnosis," June 17, 2021, https://www.medicalnewstoday.com/articles/ gender-bias-in-medical-diagnosis#how-does-it-affect-diagnosis.
4. Zia Sherrell Mph, "What Are the Symptoms of Heart Disease in Women?," February 22, 2021, https:// www.medicalnewstoday.com/articles/heart-disease-in-women#gender-bias.
5. Christina Jewett, "'I'm Scared to Death': Behind the Shortage Keeping Cancer Patients from Chemo," *New York Times*, December 19, 2023, https://www.nytimes. com/2023/12/19/health/cancer-drug-shortage.html.
6. CDC, "About PrEP," www.cdc.gov, November 3, 2020, https://www.cdc.gov/hiv/basics/prep/about-prep.html.
7. Alisa Figueroa, interview with author, September 6, 2023.

Chapter 7: Communicating with Your Doctors

1. Urânia Fernandes et al., "Breast Cancer in Young Women: A Rising Threat: A 5-year Follow-up Comparative

Study," *Porto Biomedical Journal* 8, no. 3 (May 1, 2023), https://doi.org/10.1097/j.pbj.0000000000000213.

2. American Medical Association, "Doctor Shortages Are Here—and They'll Get Worse If We Don't Act Fast," *American Medical Association*, April 13, 2022, https://www.ama-assn.org/practice-management/sustainability/doctor-shortages-are-here-and-they-ll-get-worse-if-we-don-t-act.

3. Rebekah Bernard, "Match Day 2023 a Reminder of the Real Cause of the Physician Shortage: Not Enough Residency Positions," *Medical Economics*, March 15, 2023, https://www.medicaleconomics.com/view/match-day-2023-a-reminder-of-the-real-cause-of-the-physician-shortage-not-enough-residency-positions.

4. Dr. Kristina Austin, personal interview with the author, April 11, 2023.

5. Dr. Amanda Hoover, personal interview with the author, August 11, 2023.

6. Raj Tek Sehgal and Paul Gorman, "Internal Medicine Physicians' Knowledge of Health Care Charges," *Journal of Graduate Medical Education* 3, no. 2 (June 1, 2011): 182–87, https://doi.org/10.4300/jgme-d-10-00186.1.

7. Dr. Kristina Austin, personal interview with the author, April 11, 2023.

8. Dr. Lisa Cook, personal interview with author, January 5, 2024.

9. Dr. Kristina Austin, personal interview with the author, April 11, 2023.

10. Dr. Lisa Cook, personal interview with author, January 5, 2024.

11. Hoover, Dr. Amanda, personal interview with the author, August 11, 2023.

12. Katrina Hutchison, "Epistemic Injustice and Questions of Credibility," in *Springer eBooks*, 2020, 27–35, https://doi.org/10.1007/978-3-030-43236-2_3.

13. Lisa Desjardins and Courtney Norris, "Podcast 'The Retrievals' Reveals Painful Experiences of Female Patients Are Often Ignored," *PBS News*, August 30, 2023, https://www.pbs.org/newshour/show/podcast-the-retrievals-reveals-painful-experiences-of-female-patients-are-often-ignored.

14. "'This Is What Women Go Through': An Account of Women's Pain in 'The Retrievals,'" America Magazine, August 29, 2023, https://www.americamagazine.org/arts-culture/2023/08/29/retrievals-podcast-serial-women-pain-ivf-245931.

15. Marie Vigouroux et al., "'He Told Me My Pain Was in My Head': Mitigating Testimonial Injustice Through Peer Support," *Frontiers in Pain Research* 4 (May 22, 2023), https://doi.org/10.3389/fpain.2023.1125963.

Chapter 8: What to Do If a Bill Is Wrong or Coverage Is Denied

1. US Department of Health and Human Services and Christi A. Grimm, "Some Medicare Advantage Organization Denials of Prior Authorization Requests Raise Concerns About Beneficiary Access to Medically Necessary Care," report, *U.S. Department of Health And Human Services Office of Inspector General*, April 2022, https://oig.hhs.gov/oei/reports/OEI-09-18-00260.pdf.

2. Marshall Allen, *Never Pay the First Bill: And Other Ways to Fight the Health Care System and Win* (New York: Penguin, 2021).

3. Kara Rayburn, "What Is the Difference Between an Internal and External Appeal?," Patient Empowerment Network, May 25, 2022, https://powerfulpatients. org/2022/05/25/what-is-the-difference-between-an-internal-and-external-appeal.

4. Jack Hoadley, Katie Keith, and Kevin W. Lucia, "Unpacking The No Surprises Act: An Opportunity to Protect Millions," Health Affairs Blog, December 18, 2020, https://www.healthaffairs.org/content/forefront/unpacking-no-surprises-act-opportunity-protect-millions.

5. Darius Tahir, "When a Quick Telehealth Visit Yields Multiple Surprises Beyond a Big Bill," *NPR*, December 19, 2023, https://www.npr.org/sections/health-shots/2023/12/19/1219693344/when-a-quick-telehealth-visit-yields-multiple-surprises-beyond-a-big-bill.

6. Tahir, "When a Quick Telehealth Visit Yields Multiple Surprises Beyond a Big Bill."

Chapter 9: Creative Solutions and Mindfulness

1. "What You Need to Know About Toxic Positivity," Right as Rain by UW Medicine, December 21, 2023, https://rightasrain.uwmedicine.org/mind/well-being/toxic-positivity.

2. Jeffrey M. Greeson and Gabrielle R. Chin, "Mindfulness and Physical Disease: A Concise Review," *Current Opinion in Psychology* 28 (August 1, 2019): 204–10, https://doi.org/10.1016/j.copsyc.2018.12.014.

3. Center for Mindful Psychotherapy, "Mindfulness for Chronic Illness: 9 Ways It Helps You Cope," Center for Mindful Therapy, June 8, 2022, https://mindfulcenter.org/9-ways-mindfulness-can-help-you-cope-with-chronic-illness/.

4. John Brent Forward et al., "Effect of Structured Touch and Guided Imagery," *Permanente Journal* 19, no. 4 (2015): 18–28. https://doi.org/10.7812/TPP/14-236.

5. "Mental Health Benefits of Journaling," WebMD, February 25, 2024, https://www.webmd.com/mental-health/mental-health-benefits-of-journaling.

Chapter 10: What Is the Real Problem?

1. Elisabeth Rosenthal, *An American Sickness: How Healthcare Became Big Business and how You Can Take it Back* (New York: Penguin, 2017).

2. Donald M. Berwick, "Salve Lucrum: The Existential Threat of Greed in US Health Care," *JAMA* 329, no. 8 (February 28, 2023): 629, https://doi.org/10.1001/jama.2023.0846.

3. Rebecca Lake, "Guide to the Sectors of the S&P 500 and Their Weights," SoFi Learn, May 18, 2024, https://www.sofi.com/learn/content/sp-500-sectors/.

4. Rebecca Lake, "What Are Cyclical Stocks?" SoFi Learn, October 4, 2023, https://www.sofi.com/learn/content/what-are-cyclical-stocks/.

5. John E. McDonough, "Our Greedy Health Care System," *American Journal of Public Health* 107, no. 11 (November 1, 2017): 1744–45, https://doi.org/10.2105/ajph.2017.304065.

6. Mark Schlesinger and Bradford H. Gray, "How Non-profits Matter in American Medicine, and What to Do About It," *Health Affairs* 25, no. Suppl1 (January 1, 2006): W287–303, https://doi.org/10.1377/hlthaff.25. w287.

7. Amol S. Navathe, "Opinion | Why Are Nonprofit Hospitals Focused More on Dollars than Patients?," *New York Times*, November 30, 2023, https://www. nytimes.com/2023/11/30/opinion/hospitals-nonprofit-community.html?smid=nytcore-ios-share&referring Source=articleShare.

8. Jessica Silver-Greenberg and Katie Thomas, "'They Were Entitled to Free Care. Hospitals Hounded Them to Pay.," *New York Times*, September 24, 2022, https:// www.nytimes.com/2022/09/24/business/nonprofit-hospitals-poor-patients.html.

9. Reed Abelson and Margot Sanger-Katz, "'The Cash Monster Was Insatiable': How Insurers Exploited Medicare for Billions," *New York Times*, October 8, 2022, https:// www.nytimes.com/2022/10/08/upshot/medicare-advantage-fraud-allegations.html.

10. Paige Minemyer, "CVS' Karen Lynch Was the Higher Paid Payer CEO Last Year," Fierce Healthcare, May 1, 2023, https://www.fiercehealthcare.com/special-reports/ heres-what-ceos-major-national-payers-earned-last-year.

11. Linda Girgis, "Will Corporate Greed Destroy Our Healthcare System?," *Physician's Weekly*, January 23, 2015, https://www.physiciansweekly.com/will-corporate-greed-destroy-healthcare-system/.

12. Frances C. Roberts, "Dopesick: Dealers, Doctors, and the Drug Company That Addicted America, by Beth Macy," *Baylor University Medical Center Proceedings* 32,

no. 3 (May 17, 2019): 466–67, https://doi.org/10.1080
/08998280.2019.1589894.

13. Medha Singh and Manas Mishra, "Eli Lilly, Novo Nordisk Get Growth Stock Status on Weight-Loss Drug
Boost," *Reuters*, February 20, 2024, https://www.reuters.
com/business/healthcare-pharmaceuticals/eli-lilly-
novo-nordisk-get-growth-stock-status-weight-loss-
drug-boost-2024-02-16/.

14. US Department of Health and Human Services and
Christi A. Grimm, "Some Medicare Advantage
Organization Denials of Prior Authorization Requests
Raise Concerns About Beneficiary Access to Medically
Necessary Care," report, *U.S. Department of Health
And Human Services Office of Inspector General*, April
2022, https://oig.hhs.gov/oei/reports/OEI-09-18-
00260.pdf.

15. "Never Pay the First Bill," Marshall Allen, n.d., https://
www.marshallallen.com/.

16. "Five Ways Commercial Insurer Policies Drive up Costs
and Hurt Patients," American Hospital Association,
May 2, 2022, https://www.aha.org/news/blog/2022-
05-02-five-ways-commercial-insurer-policies-drive-
costs-and-hurt-patients.

Chapter 11: The Safety Net

1. While this quote is attributed to Margaret Mead all over
the Internet, it has never been tied to a particular piece of
her writing, and the sleuths at Quote Investigator believe
the attribution is likely incorrect and clearly unsub-
stantiated. I like it anyway! https://quoteinvestigator.
com/2014/11/10/you-unique/#:~:text=Dear%20

Quote%20Investigator%3A%20A%20very,Just%20 like%20everyone%20else.

2. George B. Moseley, "The U.S. Health Care Non-System, 1908–2008," *The AMA Journal of Ethic* 10, no. 5 (May 1, 2008): 324–31, https://doi.org/10.1001/ virtualmentor.2008.10.5.mhst1-0805.

3. Moseley, "The U.S. Health Care Non-System, 1908–2008."

4. Moseley, "The U.S. Health Care Non-System, 1908–2008."

5. Abraham Flexner, *Medical Education in the United States and Canada: A Report to the Carnegie Foundation for the Advancement of Teaching (Classic Reprint)*, 2015.

6. "US Population: From 1900," n.d., http://demographia. com/db-uspop1900.htm.

7. Moseley, "The U.S. Health Care Non-System, 1908–2008."

8. "Indiana University Study Finds Majority of U.S. Physicians Favor National Health Insurance Support Has Grown 10 Percent Over Past 5 Years," News, April 1, 2008, https://medicine.iu.edu/news/2008/04/indiana-university-study-finds-majority-of-u-s-physicians-favor-national-health-insurance-support-has-grown-10-percent-over-past-5-years.

9. "Why The United States Has No National Health Insurance: Stakeholder Mobilization Against the Welfare State, 1945–1996," PubMed, 2004, https://pubmed. ncbi.nlm.nih.gov/15779464/.

10. Social Security Administration, Social Rehabilitation Service, and Health Care Financing Administration, "Medicare & Medicaid Milestones 1937–2015," *Medicare & Medicaid Milestones*, July 2015, https:// www.cms.gov/about-cms/agency-information/history/

downloads/medicare-and-medicaid-milestones-1937-2015.pdf.

11. Paul M. Ellwood et al., "Health Maintenance Strategy," *Medical Care* 9, no. 3 (May 1, 1971): 291–99, https://doi.org/10.1097/00005650-197105000-00008.

12. Esther Uyehara and Margaret Thomas, "*Health Maintenance Organization and the HMO Act of 1973*," RAND, Document number P-5554, 1975.

13. Moseley, "The U.S. Health Care Non-System, 1908–2008."

14. "*Medicare Hospital Prospective Payment System, How DRG Rates Are Calculated and Updated*," Office of Inspector General, August 2001, http://oig.hhs.gov/oei/reports/oei-09-00-00200.pdf.

15. Moseley, "The U.S. Health Care Non-System, 1908–2008."

16. Stephanie Armour, "The Affordable Care Act: A Brief History," *Wall Street Journal*, June 17, 2021, sec. Politics, https://www.wsj.com/articles/the-affordable-care-act-a-brief-history-11623961600.

17. "Health Coverage Protects You From High Medical Costs," HealthCare.gov, n.d., https://www.healthcare.gov/why-coverage-is-important/protection-from-high-medical-costs/.

18. "Health Coverage Protects You From High Medical Costs."

19. Jean Yi, "More States Are Proposing Single-Payer Health Care. Why Aren't They Succeeding?," *FiveThirtyEight*, March 9, 2022, https://fivethirtyeight.com/features/more-states-are-proposing-single-payer-health-care-why-arent-they-succeeding/.

20. Yi, "More States Are Proposing Single-Payer Health Care. Why Aren't They Succeeding?"

Conclusion: We Can Make This Better for Women

1. Goldsbury, Amy, private interview with author, September 5, 2023.
2. "NIH, Women's Health Initiative," Nih.gov, May 5, 2014, https://www.nhlbi.nih.gov/science/womens-health-initiative-whi; CDC, "Women's Health," https://www.cdc.gov/womens-health/index.html.
3. Go Red for Women, https://www.goredforwomen.org/en/.